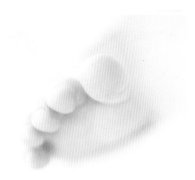

pregnancy
companion

SYDNEY ULTRASOUND *for* WOMEN

Published by Murdoch Books Pty Ltd.
©Text Sydney Ultrasound for Women. Website: www.sufw.com.au
©Design and illustrations Murdoch Books 2003. All rights reserved.
First published 2003. Reprinted 2004, 2005, 2006.

Chief Executive: Juliet Rogers
Publisher: Kay Scarlett

Creative Director: Marylouise Brammer
Designer: Vivien Valk
Photography: Sue Stubbs
Photography in inset on back cover and on pages 6–7, 16–17, 58–9, 102–3,
148–9, 176–7, 186–7: Joe Filshie
Editorial Director: Diana Hill
Editor: Sarah Baker

National Library of Australia Cataloguing-in-Publication Data
    Pregnancy companion.
    Includes index.
    ISBN 1 74045 045 0.
    1. Pregnancy. 2. Childbirth. I. Anderson, Jock. II. Stubbs, Sue.
    618.2

Produced by Phoenix Offset. PRINTED IN CHINA.

Murdoch Books Australia
Pier 8/9, 23 Hickson Road
Millers Point NSW 2000
Telephone: +61 (2) 8220 2000
Fax: +61 (2) 8220 2558

Murdoch Books UK Ltd
Erico House, 6th Floor North
93/99 Upper Richmond Road
Putney, London SW15 2TG
Telephone: +44 (0) 20 8785 5995
Fax: +44 (0) 20 8785 5985

The publisher would like to thank the following for supplying products for photography.

Bodywise Underwear, Phone (02) 9361 6052 for the maternity bras (p. 81); **Corban & Blair**, 2 Victoria Street, Lewisham
NSW 2049, Phone (02) 9560 0122 and **Childsmart/Promark Marketing** childsmart ,164 Hargrave Street, Paddington
NSW 2021, Phone (02) 9328 0488 for the baby's journal (cover, pp. 5, 185); **Funkis Swedish Forms**, 23c Curlewis Street,
Bondi NSW 2026, Phone (02) 9130 6445 for the natural brushes (p. 87), duck brush (p. 183); **Humble Beginnings**, 209
Avoca Road, Randwick NSW 2031, Phone (02) 9326 4383 for the pyjamas, slippers, toiletry bag (pp. 4, 136–7), address
book (pp. 5, 55), make-up bag (pp. 5, 167), baby socks (pp. 5, 185), pillow (pp. 40, 42–3), baby blanket (pp. 128–9), bib
(p. 147), nightie (pp. 154–5), baby bag (p. 166); **Pigott's Store**, 53 Ocean Street, Woollahra NSW 2025, Phone (02) 9362
8119 for the cup, saucer and napkins (pp. 4, 72), crockery and napkins (pp. 74–5); **Teedee Teddybears** for the teddy bear
(pp. 65, 181); **The Baby's Ark**, 81–85 Frenchmans Road, North Randwick NSW 2031, Phone (02) 9326 5036 and **Ark
Homewares**, 79 Frenchmans Road, North Randwick NSW 2031, Phone (02) 9314 5755 for the bassinet and stand, pillow
(pp. 128–9); **The Parterre Garden**, 33 Ocean Street, Woollahra NSW 2025, Phone (02) 9363 5874 for the basin (p. 31).

Photograph on p. 21 of fertilisation of egg by sperm and photograph on p. 53 of fetus at 12 weeks: photolibrary.com

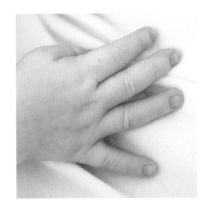

pregnancy companion

Dr John C Anderson

Dr Tom Boogert

Dr Greg J Kesby

Dr Andrew C McLennan

Ms Janette O'Connor

Dr Robert D Robertson

Dr Fergus P Scott

MURDOCH
B O O K S

contents

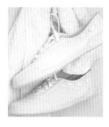
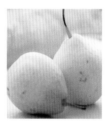
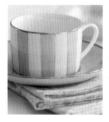
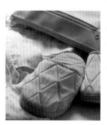

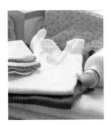

after the birth

Here's what to expect from the first six weeks of motherhood, from the joy of the birth to adjusting to your new role

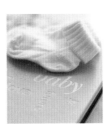

baby's journal

Record the details of your baby's birth, developmental milestones and christening or naming ceremony

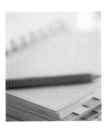

helpful information

Consult this section for a list of commonly used medical terms and a directory of support groups

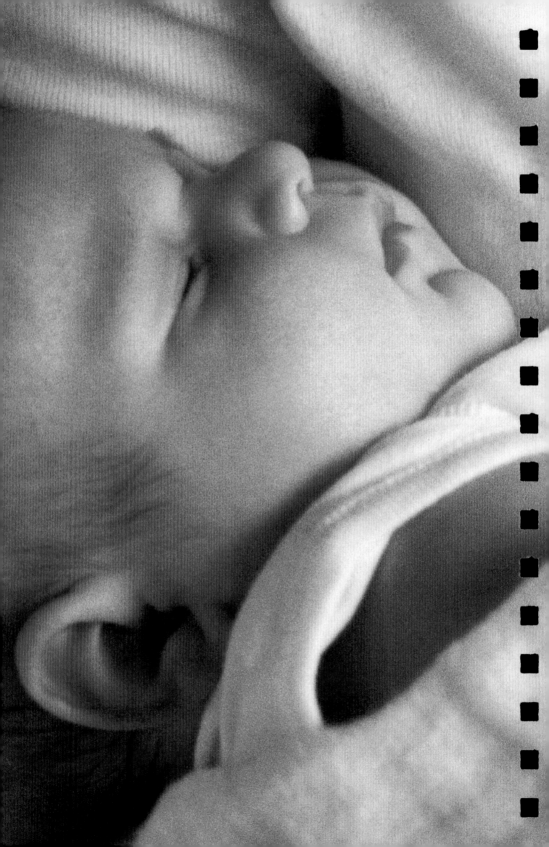

planning ahead

you've just made one of the most important decisions of your life — you're going to try for a baby! You will want to do everything possible to have a perfectly healthy one. In addition to the advice you receive from your doctor, the following suggestions may make a difference. But don't worry if your pregnancy is not planned. Many pregnancies start out this way and nature seems to do a pretty good job anyway.

preparing yourself Giving life to another human being is a joyful event in any woman's life. These days, with the development of reliable methods of contraception, it's possible to plan the timing of your pregnancy so that you're prepared in every way for the changes that a new baby will bring.

Of course, not all pregnancies are planned. Sometimes we can be caught quite offguard, but after the initial shock has passed the excitement and thrill take over. We have come a long way from the days when women gave birth at home, often with only another woman in attendance. You have the advantage of advanced medical care and the choice of many support groups, ranging from antenatal (before delivery) to postnatal (after delivery). You will find a list of some of these support groups on page 189.

your medical history

If you are planning a pregnancy, go and see your family doctor first for advice and a general check-up. He may identify specific risk factors from your or your partner's family or personal history, your physical examination or from additional laboratory testing which he may have arranged. These factors may affect your health or your baby's during pregnancy.

If you suffer from a pre-existing medical condition such as asthma, diabetes, hypertension or depression, you may be taking medication. If that is the case, you should obtain expert advice about becoming pregnant while on medication; it may be that changing the prescription medicine will be safer for the baby.

If you are an older woman (over 35), or if there is a family history of a birth defect, genetic problem or intellectual disability, your doctor may refer you to a specialist for genetic counselling. The history, examination and specific laboratory tests obtained may help to determine your risk of having an affected baby. Your options for testing during pregnancy will also be discussed.

Your doctor will want to confirm that you have immunity to rubella (German measles), and will vaccinate you if you don't. There is an 80 per cent risk of serious birth defects — including heart defects, deafness and cataracts — if a pregnant woman who has no immunity to rubella is infected during the first trimester. Last, but not least, you will be advised to take folic acid supplementation to reduce the risk of having a baby with spina bifida. You must take this for three months prior to the intended time of conception and for the first three months of pregnancy.

Once your doctor has given you the green light, it's up to you and your partner. You may not conceive straightaway. In fact it may take a healthy couple up to 12 months to conceive. During this time you need to remain well, get adequate rest, take regular exercise and eat a balanced diet.

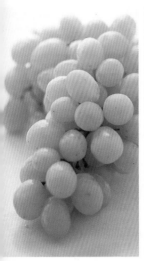

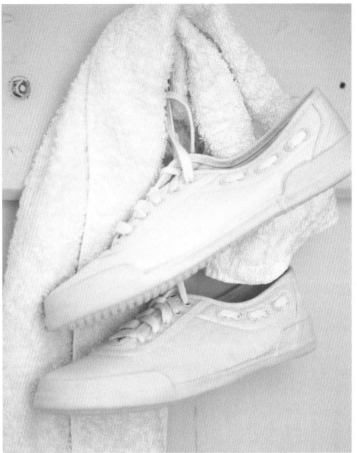

exercise and diet For regular exercise, choose an activity that you enjoy. It may be walking or swimming. It may be going to the gym, but make sure you seek guidance from a qualified instructor once you become pregnant. It's best to avoid contact sports during your pregnancy.

Preparing your body for pregnancy is an important part of the planning process. Your diet should be balanced, with foods and nutrients that will benefit you and your baby. These include protein, iron, complex carbohydrates, calcium, zinc, vitamin C, vitamin B12, vitamin D, folic acid, omega 3 fatty acids and plenty of water. Check out which foods you like that contain these building blocks and nutrients (see the table on page 26).

You should increase your intake of folate (or folic acid) at least one month before becoming pregnant (preferably three months) and into the early months of pregnancy. Folic acid is found in fresh fruit and vegetables, legumes, cereals and bread, and supplements are available from your chemist.

Calcium, for the development of strong teeth and bones, is also necessary, as are omega 3 fatty acids, found in cold-water fish. Omega 3s help to prevent inflammation, influence baby's vision and assist in maintaining a healthy heart.

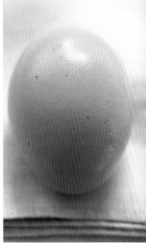

what to avoid
Foods to avoid include blue cheeses, liver pâté, unpasteurised goat's milk or cheese, and undercooked meat. There is a risk of listeria with the first two and toxoplasmosis with the others. Listeria infection during pregnancy may cause miscarriage. Toxoplasmosis infection during pregnancy involves a low risk for fetal brain damage and blindness.

Drink no more than one or two units of alcohol once or twice a week (one unit is equivalent to a small glass of wine). The harmful effects to the baby of excessive amounts of alcohol include mental retardation, behavioural problems and major birth defects. If you choose to drink alcohol, dilute it by drinking lots of other fluids. Limit caffeine to no more than 150 mg (0.0154 grain) per day (equivalent to two cups of instant coffee, tea or cola). Give up smoking cigarettes and using recreational drugs, as they are harmful to the baby. Smoking may cause a baby to be born with a low birth weight and an increased risk for cot death. Avoid taking retinol, which is a form of vitamin A. It is present in some acne treatments and has been linked to birth defects. Also avoid spas as they cause overheating of the body. And wear gloves when gardening or handling the cat's litter: both garden soil and cat's litter can cause toxoplasmosis.

It's best to be cautious but optimistic when planning ahead for a baby. If in doubt about anything, always ask your doctor.

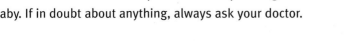

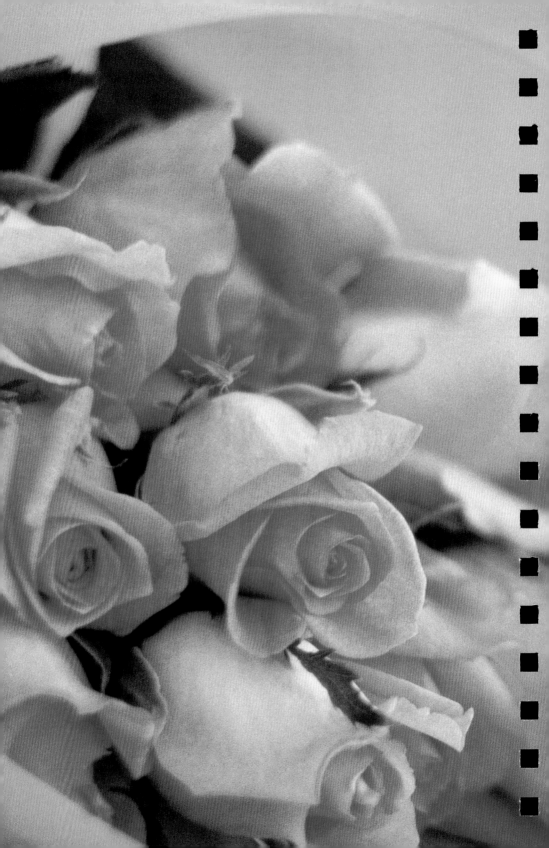

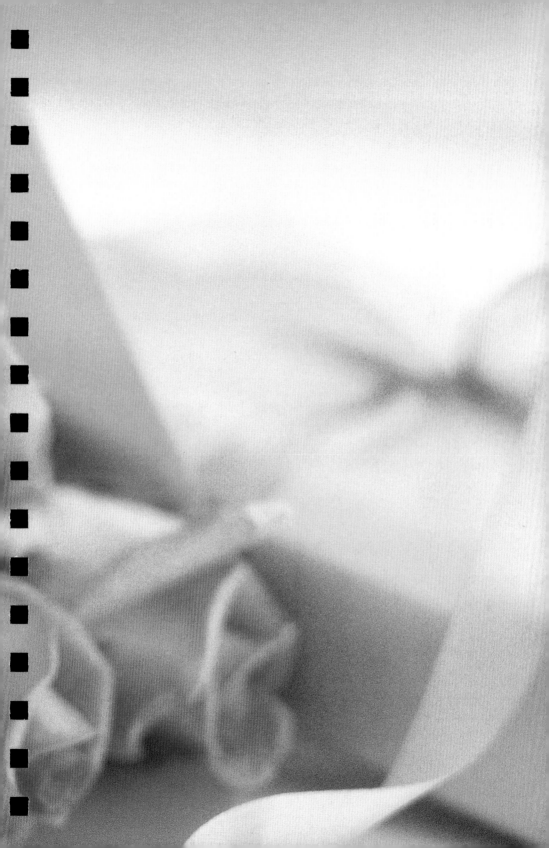

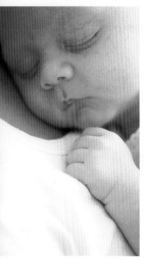

planning your pregnancy
If you and your partner decide to start a family, there are certain matters you should consider.

Maternity leave

You'll need to decide if you intend to return to work after having the baby, and if so, how much maternity leave you should take. If you are not aware of the maternity leave conditions offered by your employer, speak to your boss or human resources manager.

Check how many weeks' notice you need to give your employer; you may also be asked to provide proof of pregnancy. Keep in touch with your employer from time to time while you are on maternity leave.

Financial planning

It's a good idea to sit down with your partner and draw up a budget, listing your income, living costs and commitments. This will show if you can cope with one salary, even for a few months. Actually try to live on one salary for a while to see if it is possible.

Another option is to see your bank manager and let her know what you are planning. If you own your own home, ask her to discuss your mortgage's fine print with you and if the repayments can be restructured for the period you intend to be away from work. You could also consult a financial planner. This can be an expensive exercise, so ask what costs you will be liable for before you receive any advice.

Newborn babies can be very expensive. There are many items you need to buy, particularly in the first few weeks after birth. Some mothers, who only went to the chemist a few times a year before having a baby, find themselves there weekly, sometimes daily, after their baby's arrival! Make sure you have some savings put aside as these chemist trips can be devastating to a household budget.

CONCEIVING

Be prepared for the event that you may not fall pregnant immediately. It may take a few months to conceive, and age is a predisposing factor: the older you get, the longer it can take to fall pregnant. There are no hard and fast rules though.

Running your own business

If you are self-employed then you know that running a business can be very time-consuming. If you can afford it, consider employing a manager for the last month of your pregnancy and for the first three months after the birth. The expense may be worth the peace of mind this provides so that you can enjoy this time with your baby. The manager may be able to stay on part-time after this period, allowing you the flexibility of shorter hours for as long you need it.

If you are an accountant, doctor or lawyer, or are employed in any position where matters can become protracted, review your case load and keep a colleague involved to ensure a smooth handover when you leave work.

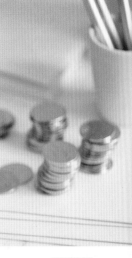

Medical insurance

Take the time to visit your health insurance office and ask them to explain your coverage to you clearly. Tell the representative that you are intending to have a baby and want to be sure of your entitlements.

Are you covered for obstetrics? Are you covered for a private or public hospital? Are you covered for a private or shared room? Are you covered for theatre costs? Can you have the doctor of your choice? Also ascertain how long you need to be in a particular plan to qualify for obstetric cover. It can be very disappointing to discover, after you have fallen pregnant, that you do not have sufficient medical insurance cover to have your baby where and how you want.

SAVINGS
There are bound to be some unforeseen expenses in the course of your pregnancy. If you're wise, you'll devise a sensible savings plan as soon as you can.

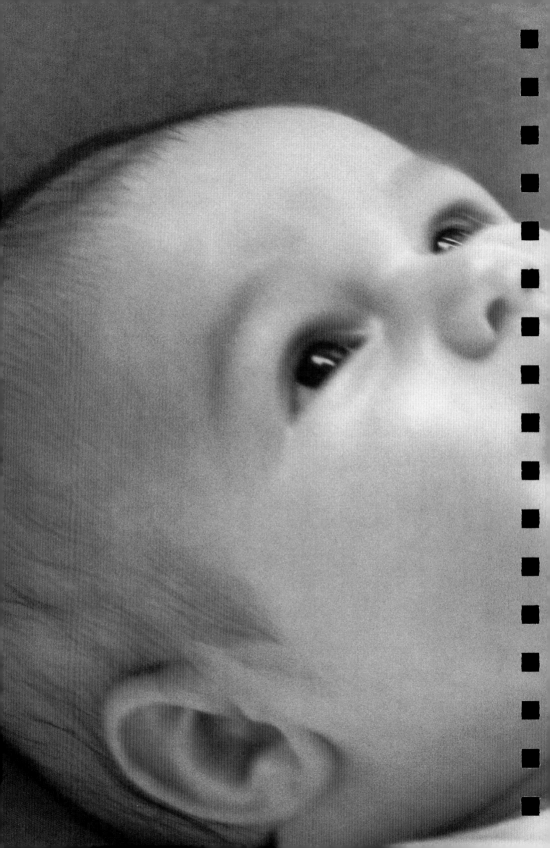

first trimester

having a baby, particularly for the first time, is one of the great milestones in a woman's life. It is a truly wonderful experience. Enjoy every step. Be amazed by every change taking place within your body as you feel the little person grow inside you.

week 1

DATE 05 : 06 · 14

you

the gestation of a human pregnancy is nine months. That is 38 weeks when we consider that most months are not 28 days but 30 or 31 days. To confuse matters more, your health professional will talk about 40 weeks of pregnancy.

Believe it or not, there is a very good reason for choosing to make the whole episode two weeks longer. It is important to elect a starting date. A woman usually ovulates 14 days before her *next* menstrual period. If she becomes pregnant there is no *next* menstrual period, so the easiest date to pinpoint is the first day of the *last* menstrual period (LMP). From that date we can calculate that a woman with a 28-day cycle will ovulate on day 14 of that cycle. Therefore day 1 of week 1 is the first day of your last menstrual period, and day 14 is the day you ovulate. In fact, you haven't even conceived until two weeks into your 'pregnancy'.

So the LMP is a useful way to calculate the estimated date of delivery (EDD). If your cycle is not a regular 28-day cycle, then the LMP method is less accurate. Should you have a very erratic cycle or are unsure of the date of your LMP, an early ultrasound is the most accurate method of establishing the EDD.

The average normal human pregnancy lasts for 283 days, or 40 weeks and three days. Conventionally it has been divided into three trimesters. The first trimester is from week 1 to week 13. The second trimester includes weeks 14 to 26, and the third trimester is from week 27 to week 40, or whenever you have the baby. A pregnancy rarely goes past 42 weeks.

While the first week of your cycle may sound relatively mundane, lots of things happen that are important to the success of your impending pregnancy. The lining of your womb or uterus is shed

week 1

during menstruation; this serves as a type of spring-cleaning. Your uterus is now ready to start building up its lining again in preparation for the 'planting' of the fertilised egg or ovum. This process happens during every single cycle.

week 2

you

on the last day of this week you will ovulate. But there's a lot more to it than that. Each ovary has numerous 'follicles' close to its surface. Each follicle is a little cyst containing an egg, which grows on the inside of its wall. The follicles all start to develop at different rates under the influence of hormones made by the pituitary gland at the base of the brain. As the follicles develop, a sort of internal hormonal struggle occurs in the ovaries as each follicle attempts to suppress its neighbours. One will eventually increase in size faster than the others; this follicle becomes known as the 'dominant' follicle.

Occasionally there is a slip-up and two 'dominant' follicles develop simultaneously, resulting in twins. Twins occurring from ovulations such as this are as genetically different as brothers and sisters from separate pregnancies, so they are known as non-identical twins. Rarely, when only one egg is fertilised, identical twins can be produced. This happens after the cell divides into two or more cells and they subsequently split, continuing to grow separately. Each has the same chromosomal and genetic make-up, so they are identical.

The egg nestled inside the dominant follicle contains the full complement of your genetic material, mapped or encoded on 46 chromosomes grouped into 23 pairs, one of which came from your father and the other from your mother. A process called meiosis then occurs: the chromosomes double, and then divide twice, retaining only half of their genetic material (that is, 23 chromosomes). This step must be perfect for the egg to have the correct number and structure of chromosomes.

All the eggs you will ever have are in your ovaries when you are born, therefore as you grow older, so do your eggs. Because the

FIRST TRIMESTER

energy in the egg decreases over time, this process sometimes goes wrong and leaves an incorrect number of chromosomes in the egg, resulting in a chromosomally abnormal pregnancy. For instance, an extra chromosome in the number 21 group results in Down syndrome. Although these errors occur regularly, most of these eggs remain unfertilised, or if fertilised, pass out of the body without implanting. This means the vast majority of all ongoing pregnancies are chromosomally normal.

Before ovulation the dominant follicle reaches 20–24 mm (0.8–0.9 in) in diameter. The egg and the surrounding fluid are released into the abdominal cavity. The egg is enticed towards the fallopian tube by soft finger-like projections, called fimbria, on the end of the tube. Situated close to the ovary, they create a wafting motion, assisting the egg down the tube. The follicle in which the egg originated has now collapsed. It produces estrogen and progesterone, which instruct the lining of the uterus to thicken. Conception is most likely to occur from day 14–17 in a regular 28-day cycle.

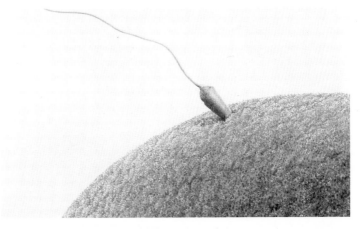

A SPERM FERTILISING AN EGG

DATE ....

you

as your egg wafts down the fallopian tube, the sperm swim upwards in a (usually) vain and glorious attempt to be *the* one. That one sperm will re-create itself in the form of another human. First the sperm swims up through the cervix, then on through the uterine cavity, finally meeting with your egg in the fallopian tube. It may take one to three days for the sperm and ovum to meet, so the date of intercourse is not always the date of conception.

A tough clear shell called the zona pellucida protects the egg. The sperm has a special 'hat' on its head called an acrosome, which has the ability to stick to the zona pellucida and then to dissolve a little tunnel in it, allowing it to enter the egg. It then swims a short distance to the soft egg itself and enters, carrying its genetic material in a little package called a pronucleus. The genetic material in the egg is also contained in a pronucleus so now there are two pronuclei.

Girls have two X chromosomes (XX) and boys have an X and a Y chromosome (XY). The pronucleus in the egg always carries an X chromosome, never a Y. A sperm can carry an X or Y chromosome. Therefore, if the pronucleus from the sperm carries a Y chromosome, the baby will be a boy, and if it carries an X chromosome, the baby will be a girl.

If the fertilised egg remains in the fallopian tube and implants there, it will become an ectopic pregnancy. Fortunately, ectopic pregnancies are rare. An ectopic pregnancy is dangerous because it can rupture, causing severe internal bleeding.

The embryo passes along the fallopian tube and develops into a solid ball of cells, then enters the uterine cavity on day 4 after conception. It floats freely from day 5 to day 8, then implants on day 9–12. By this time it is a 'blastocyst', which means it has cells surrounding a cystic area. The pregnancy is still very small and is not visible on ultrasound.

The lining of your uterus has become thicker, secreting a lot of nutritious fluid, which makes it capable of accepting an embryo for implantation. Later the pregnancy produces a hormone called hCG (human chorionic gonadotrophin), which acts on the old follicle (now called a corpus luteum), allowing it to produce more estrogen and progesterone. hCG is the hormone used in pregnancy tests and will later be found in increasing levels in both your blood and your urine. Pregnancy tests are not usually positive until week 4.

Many conceptions do not have a correct complement of genetic material (chromosomes) and are unable to survive. This accounts for the very high miscarriage rate in early pregnancy. It has been estimated that 2 out of 3 of all conceptions will miscarry. Once a pregnancy has been confirmed, more than 85 per cent of babies will survive to birth.

During this early stage the placenta has not yet formed and is not able to take nutrients from your circulation; instead nutrients are taken from the fluid surrounding the early pregnancy. At this point any insult to the pregnancy tends to have an all or nothing effect: either the pregnancy miscarries or it is unaffected.

Occasionally a woman may be x-rayed in early pregnancy before she even realises she is pregnant, and no precautions, such as covering the abdomen with a lead apron, are taken. Usually no detrimental effect is seen, even if the x-ray was in the abdominal region, because the fetus's organs are not forming at this stage.

week 4

you

at this time you would expect your next menstrual period if you hadn't conceived. You may experience some bleeding, although it won't be as heavy as a normal period. This bleeding is due to the implantation process, where the pregnancy buries into the lining of the uterus. Many women falsely believe that this light bleeding indicates that they are not pregnant, resulting in the dating for the pregnancy being incorrect by four weeks.

The changes you normally experience before a period, such as breast tenderness, continue. However, your breasts continue to enlarge and become even more sensitive. This is often the first outward sign of pregnancy, confirming that the small amount of bleeding was not a real period. As each day passes without a period, the possibility of a long menstrual cycle decreases and the probability of a pregnancy increases. It is around this time that pregnancy tests start to become positive. The hormone hCG can be detected at very low levels in your blood and the latest versions of the urine pregnancy test are able to detect it.

MY WEIGHT _____

MY BELLY WIDTH _____

APPOINTMENTS _____

your baby

the cystic structure (blastocyst) is rapidly growing and soon some of the cells start to become the embryonic disc. This will continue to develop and, in time, will become the fetus. The fluid-filled area becomes the amniotic cavity in which the fetus lives. The placental tissue grows and invades the lining of your uterus, much like a plant sending roots into the earth; it establishes an interface with your circulation. Your vessels in the region of the placenta dilate to supply more blood to the developing pregnancy. The pregnancy is still microscopic and cannot be seen on ultrasound. Only the thickened lining of the uterus is visible.

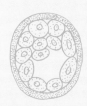

EARLY BLASTOCYST

what to eat

A healthy balanced diet will give your baby all the nutrition it needs and will also help you to keep your weight under control during pregnancy. Try to avoid fast foods, which are high in fat and salt, although an occasional take-away won't hurt. You'll need a higher intake of calcium, iron, protein and some vitamins than you would normally. Include foods from the categories listed below.

Intake	Foods
Calcium	Milk, hard cheese, yoghurt, almonds, vegetables
Iron	Chicken, fish, lean red meat, kidney beans, cereals, eggs, rice, wholegrain bread, baked beans, spinach, pasta, dried fruit
Protein	Lean red meat, chicken, beans, hard cheese
Folate	Green vegetables, soy beans, cereals, bananas
Complex carbohydrates	Fresh fruit and vegetables, cereals, nuts, pasta, potatoes, rice
Vitamin C	Citrus, capsicum (peppers), strawberries, kiwi fruit
Vitamin B12	Lean red meat, dairy foods, chicken, fish
Vitamin D	Canned fish, milk, eggs
Omega 3 fatty acids	Salmon, herring, sardines, seeds, almonds
Water	Drink at least 8 glasses a day
Zinc	Meat, peas

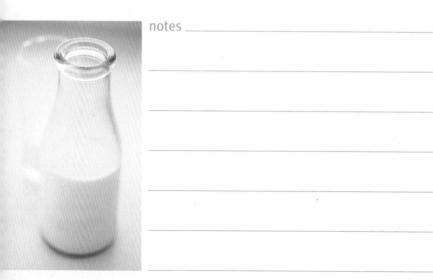

notes _____

_____

_____

_____

_____

_____

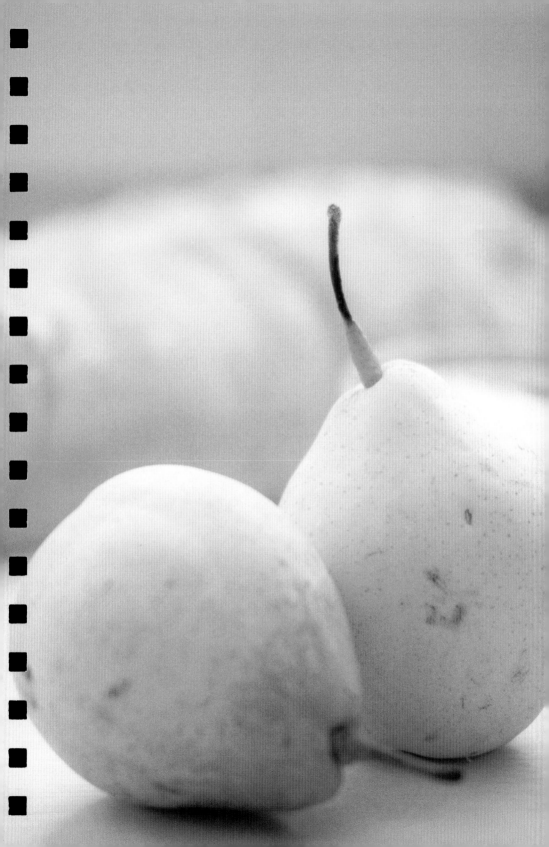

DATE ....

you

your menstrual period is now late and it is becoming more likely that there is an ongoing pregnancy rather than just a late period. The hormonal changes due to the pregnancy are just beginning. The level of hCG produced by the placental cells is increasing rapidly, doubling every two days. Once the level is above 1000 Iμ/mL, the pregnancy can usually be seen on ultrasound.

At the beginning of this week only a gestation sac can be seen (see below). This contains the yolk sac and the developing fetus. The yolk sac generally disappears by 12 weeks, having fulfilled its function of supporting the very early fetus.

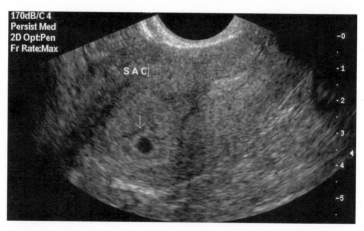

GESTATION SAC AT 5 WEEKS. A FETAL ECHO IS NOT YET SEEN

MY WEIGHT   _____

MY BELLY WIDTH   _____

APPOINTMENTS   _____

your baby

towards the end of the fifth week your baby will become visible on ultrasound. At first it just looks like a blob on the screen, but once it reaches 5 mm (0.2 in) in length, a heartbeat can be seen. This will be slow at first, then rapidly increasing to around 180 beats per minute at nine weeks.

The presence of a heartbeat is definite proof of an ongoing pregnancy. The risk of miscarriage has reduced enormously, with around 90 per cent of pregnancies likely to survive to birth. Some couples are keen to tell their friends and family about the pregnancy straightaway, while others prefer to wait a little longer, until the miscarriage rate is even lower and further tests have shown the baby to be developing normally.

Measurements
Babies grow at different rates during pregnancy. The figures quoted for lengths and weights throughout this book are therefore crude approximations only. Baby's length is the distance from the top of the head to the tip of the bottom (also called the crown rump length, or CRL). The measurement of the CRL can be used to determine the age of the baby accurately to within three days, which is very useful if the LMP is uncertain or your menstrual cycle was irregular.

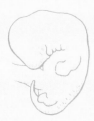

5 WEEK FETUS

pregnancy test

If your period is two weeks overdue, you can purchase a pregnancy test from your chemist and use it in the privacy of your own home, or you can make an appointment with your family doctor to confirm your pregnancy. If a positive result is shown on the home test, you will still need to see your doctor to confirm the pregnancy.

morning sickness

At around this time, the hormones from the pregnancy will start to cause some of those common side effects of pregnancy. Suddenly you cannot bear the smell of coffee, let alone the drink itself. You wake up with a 'hung-over' feeling. Yes, this is morning sickness. Unfortunately, the majority of mothers experience morning sickness during the first trimester. It can occur at any time of day, not just in the morning. It usually recedes by the second trimester.

As morning sickness is thought to be exacerbated by low blood sugar, try regulating your diet by eating little and often. Eat dry biscuits or toast in bed in the morning: ask your partner to spoil you a little with breakfast in bed. Snack on things like crackers and dried fruit. And take some ginger tablets or drink some ginger tea, as ginger is reputed to reduce nausea. Place a piece of fresh ginger root in a cup of hot water and allow it to infuse as you would a tea, then sweeten it to taste before drinking. If you don't like ginger tea, try some peppermint tea instead.

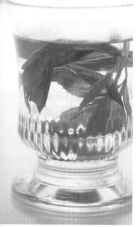

As the nausea and vomiting continue, you may be concerned that your baby is not receiving enough nutrition. There is no need to worry because the baby is very good at taking exactly what it needs to develop properly, even if it is at your expense. For this reason, eating more of what the baby needs simply replenishes your own stores of important nutrients such as calcium and iron.

If you suffer from long periods of vomiting or your morning sickness is severe, contact your obstetrician or antenatal clinic.

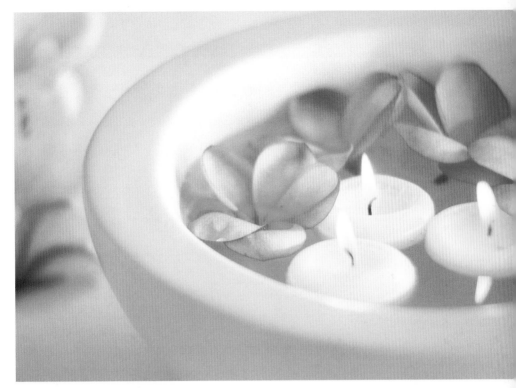

food cravings

food cravings You may experience cravings for certain foods, although not everyone wants pickled onions and ice cream. Your senses of taste and smell can alter too: certain foods that you used to enjoy now seem repulsive. Coffee and wine tend to be high on this list. Naturally, nausea and other changes are likely to diminish your libido.

your partner

your partner Although you are noticing enormous changes in your body and moods, your partner is not able to experience them. Discussing your feelings about these changes can help your partner to appreciate what is happening to you and be more understanding of shifts in your mood, behaviour, energy and libido.

TIME TOGETHER

A special meal together, whether you have it at home or in a restaurant, gives you both a chance to talk over the changes you are experiencing.

DATE . . . .

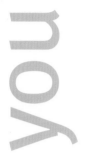

the hormonal changes continue rapidly. You may start to really feel pregnant by experiencing the tiredness that is a classic symptom of early pregnancy. Some women feel as if they have been infected with a sleeping disorder, only to be greeted by the ongoing nausea when they wake. The same hormones that cause emotional changes during the menstrual cycle are acting at much higher levels during pregnancy, so don't be surprised if you feel very emotional for no apparent reason.

Relaxin is a hormone produced by the corpus luteum. Your relaxin levels are higher during the early stages of pregnancy compared to the later ones. Relaxin causes the ligaments to have more 'give', enabling a large range of movement in most joints. This allows the ligaments holding the pelvic bones to stretch, resulting in a wider opening for the baby to pass through. But that is still many months away and, in the meantime, joints between the vertebrae in the back can move more than usual. The movement can sometimes be enough to cause some pressure on nerves. The pain is usually more severe later in the pregnancy, when the enlarging womb alters your posture.

MY WEIGHT

MY BELLY WIDTH

APPOINTMENTS

APPROXIMATELY 241 DAYS TO GO

your baby is approximately 5–10 mm (0.2–0.4 in) from head to bottom at the start of the sixth week and still looks like a blob on ultrasound. Many couples who have seen their baby at this early stage refer to it as their 'bean' due to the shape they see. Although the numerous changes in the structure cannot be seen, the heartbeat is obvious, beating at about 100 beats per minute. This is already quicker than the maternal heart rate, but it will become much quicker in the weeks to come.

The spine has been completing its development, and by day 27 after conception both ends of the spine close over. Many factors can affect the development of the spine, the best known being folic acid (folate). There appear to be other vitamins that are co-factors in spinal development and recently multivitamins, rather than just folate, have been suggested.

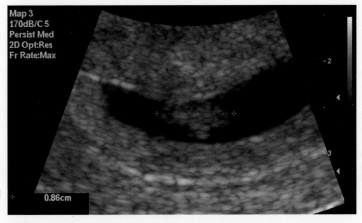

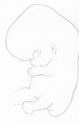

LEFT: FETUS AT 6 WEEKS. ABOVE: THE FETAL ECHO LOOKS LIKE A SMALL WHITE BLOB OR 'BEAN' IN A BLACK AMNIOTIC SAC

week 7

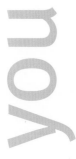

your breasts have continued to increase in size and the nipples are also undergoing change. They tend to become larger, more pigmented and erectile. The increase in breast size is mostly due to proliferation of glandular tissue, whereas later in the pregnancy the ductal tissue of the breast will proliferate.

The placenta is starting to function and is producing more than just the hormone hCG. Progesterone levels increase; among other things, progesterone is thought to cause relaxation of 'smooth muscle', which is found in the bowel and the uterus. This is one of the causes of constipation in pregnancy.

The placenta also produces a hormone called human placental lactogen (hPL). This causes resistance in your own natural insulin. As the levels of hPL rise, the ability to cope with sugars decreases. Gestational diabetes occurs when the insulin resistance during pregnancy becomes enough to warrant a change in diet to maintain lower and more normal blood sugar levels. It is rare for insulin to be required and the ability to handle sugars will return to normal after the birth of the baby.

Fluid retention is a common side effect of pregnancy. This causes an increase in your weight, which seems to have little correlation with the outcome of the pregnancy. Thus many obstetricians have stopped weighing their pregnant patients at each visit.

MY WEIGHT

MY BELLY WIDTH

APPOINTMENTS   feeling very nauseas

FIRST TRIMESTER

week 7

APPROXIMATELY 234 DAYS TO GO

your baby is approximately 1 cm (0.4 in) long by the start of the seventh week. The bean shape continues and the heart rate has increased further, to around 140 beats per minute.

your baby

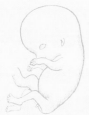

7 WEEK FETUS

notes _____

the right obstetrician

This is a good time to consider where you would like to have your baby and to choose both the hospital or birth centre and the obstetrician or midwife.

If you are covered by private medical insurance, you can choose your own obstetrician (the specialist who delivers the baby). Your family doctor may have some suggestions but you do not have to consult the obstetrician he suggests. You may already have a gynecologist/obstetrician whom you like.

Choosing the obstetrician who is best for you will depend on a few factors. You will find that obstetricians only deliver babies at certain hospitals. If you have your heart set on delivering at a particular hospital, ring the hospital and ask for a list of obstetricians who deliver at that hospital. Speak to friends who already have children and ask if they were happy with their obstetrician and why. You might prefer a female obstetrician.

Once you have chosen an obstetrician, make an appointment as soon as possible. Popular obstetricians tend to be heavily booked: if he or she has an optimum number of patients due for delivery at the same time as you, you may need to choose another doctor. Also, some tests, such as nuchal translucency at 11–13 weeks, are carried out early in pregnancy, so you need to see your obstetrician before this time (see 'Week 12'). Failing that, your family doctor can order the test and forward the results to your obstetrician.

In the end, you may find that, for one reason or another, you don't like the obstetrician you have selected. If this is the case, find another one. A good relationship with your practitioner is very important.

Make sure you reconfirm your hospital or birth centre booking a few weeks after the initial booking, just to be on the safe side.

DATE 08.02.09

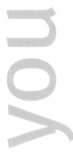

your pregnancy is small and not yet using much extra oxygen; however, the hormones created by the pregnancy cause dramatic changes in you. Your heart begins to work harder, raising the volume pumped by around 50 per cent. The increased blood flow then passes through other organs, such as the kidneys, resulting in a larger urine output and causing you to go to the toilet frequently. Your body temperature has risen slightly, and with the blood vessels in your skin dilating, you feel hotter.

Deeper breathing, along with the large blood volume passing through your heart, reduces the levels of carbon dioxide in your blood. The composition of the blood changes with an increase in the proportion of red blood cells, which carry oxygen. The combination of changes in the heart, lungs and blood massively increases your body's ability to take oxygen to your pregnancy. These changes have occurred well in advance and well in excess of the pregnancy's requirements.

There have been changes to your body shape and you will quickly realise that some clothes do not fit you as well as they did before. Although it may seem too early to shop for maternity clothes, some looser fitting clothes could help.

MY WEIGHT   51 kg

MY BELLY WIDTH

APPOINTMENTS

APPROXIMATELY 227 DAYS TO GO

your baby

your baby measures about 1.6 cm (0.6 in) from head to bottom at the start of the eighth week and is beginning to be recognisable as a human being, having a head at one end when viewed on ultrasound. The limbs have begun to develop and small limb buds can also be seen. The head at this stage is as large as the rest of the baby. Many of the organ systems are already reaching their final stages of development, with only a change in size occurring during the rest of your pregnancy.

The heart rate has increased further and will be beating at around 160 beats per minute. When compared to an adult heart rate this seems incredibly quick: most adults can only achieve a similar heart rate during strenuous exercise.

weight gain The recommended weight gain during pregnancy is between 10 and 14 kg (22 and 30.9 lb). Your obstetrician or antenatal clinic will monitor your weight gain and advise you if it's too much or too little.

fatigue You may feel extremely tired in the first two months of pregnancy, when most people are unaware that you are pregnant. It's not uncommon at this stage to find yourself asleep at the table in a restaurant or at a dinner party. This fatigue can be difficult to deal with when you are at work.

Try to go to bed earlier than usual and plan a less hectic social life. If your job requires you to be on your feet for long periods of time, ask if it is possible to sit on a stool or take regular breaks, or even change your tasks during the later months of pregnancy. Some mothers choose to work right up to the 40th week, while others take a couple of weeks to organise themselves and rest before labour begins (see 'Planning your pregnancy' on page 14).

rest Take every opportunity to rest. There's an old saying: 'Don't stand when you can sit and don't sit when you can lie down.'

notes _____

_____

_____

_____

_____

_____

_____

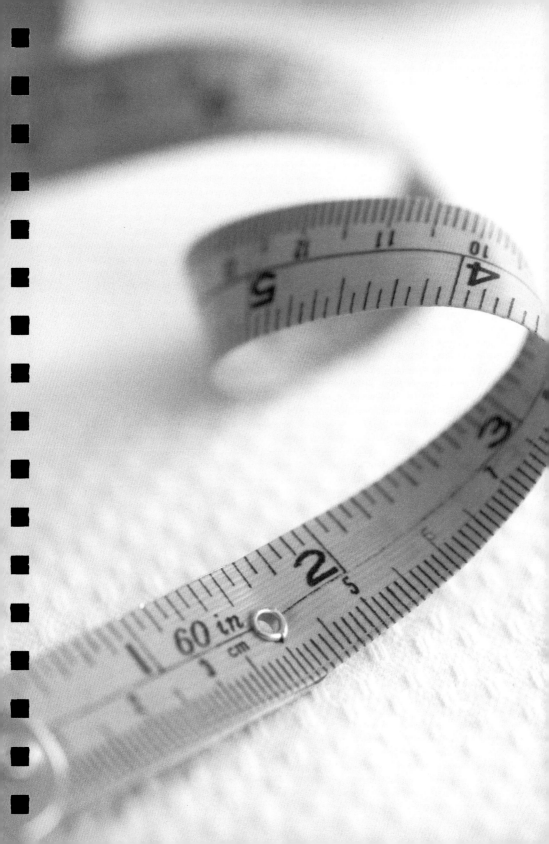

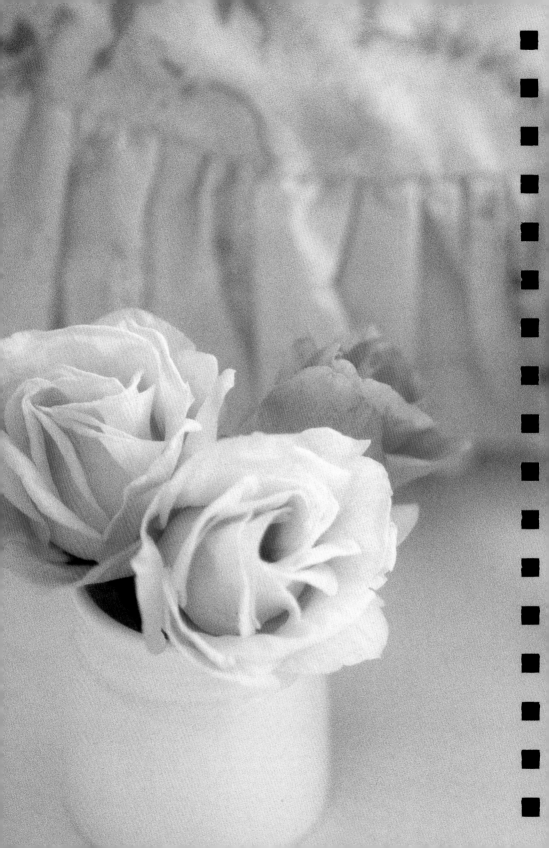

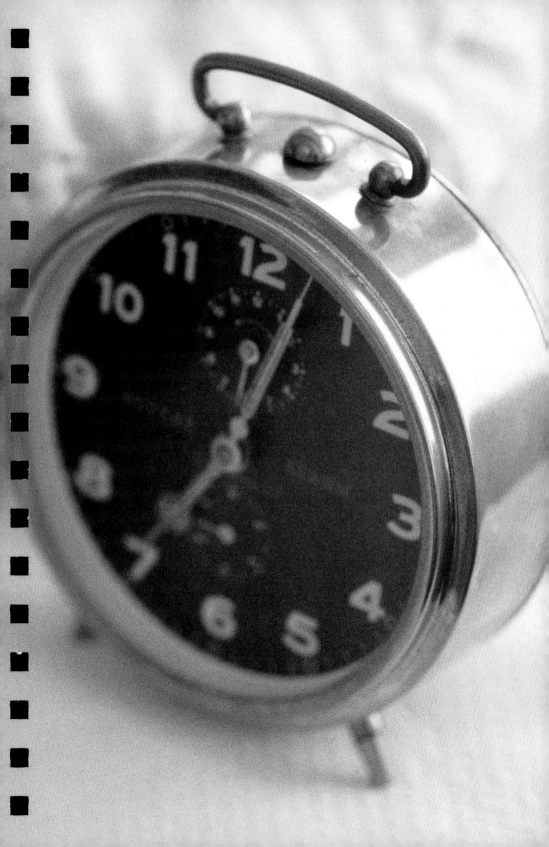

DATE 15·02·09

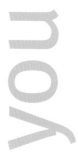

the hormonal changes due to the pregnancy
continue. Your blood pressure tends to decrease, and you may
feel lightheaded if you get up quickly or stand for extended
periods. Your face will appear flushed and warm due to the
dilation of the small blood vessels. Your facial appearance
becomes fuller due to oedema, which is due to the retention of
more fluid. An increase in the melanocyte-stimulating hormone
will enable small amounts of ultraviolet light to create a
considerable change in the amount of skin pigmentation. Hence
pregnant women usually tan extremely easily. It is important to
continue to use sun protection as you did before pregnancy, as
the risk of skin cancer is the same. Increased pigmentation on the
face is known as chloasma, or the 'mask of pregnancy'. Growth of
fine hair, called lanugo, is also stimulated at this time.

ULTRASOUND
This would be a
good time to book
your 12 week
ultrasound, which
will check that your
baby's structural
and chromosomal
development is
normal.

If you visit your doctor for a check-up at this stage, there appears
to be no end to the number of blood tests she orders. These
are useful for establishing your blood group, whether there are
any antibodies that could affect your baby, and the level of
hemoglobin to exclude anemia. Other blood tests include
checking for hepatitis, syphilis and rubella (German measles); a
urine test checking for infection will also be ordered.

MY WEIGHT

MY BELLY WIDTH

APPOINTMENTS

your baby

your baby's heart rate reaches around 180 beats per minute, as fast as the resting heart rate ever goes. This rate will continue to decrease to be about 140 beats per minute by birth and then to around 60 beats per minute as an adult. Although some people believe that the heart rate differs between male and female babies, this is usually not the case. The best way to determine the baby's gender is at 19 weeks on ultrasound, or from genetic testing. Although it is technically possible to determine the gender before birth, many couples prefer to wait and be surprised.

Your baby is almost fully developed. The arms and legs are obvious on ultrasound. The baby is able to make small movements and is really starting to look like a baby, not just a bean. It now measures 2.4 cm (0.9 in) from head to bottom.

DATE .... 22·02·09 ....

you

your uterus increases in size as the fetus and the placenta grow. At around 10 weeks the uterus is about the size of a grapefruit and can be felt through the abdomen.

At about this stage of pregnancy the risk of miscarriage is becoming very small (2–3 per cent). You may switch from worrying whether the pregnancy will continue to the end to wanting to know that your baby is normal. Although no individual test or even group of tests can determine that, some of the common problems can be excluded.

CONCERNED ABOUT SEX?

The pregnancy is not usually adversely affected by intercourse. However, some women feel more comfortable avoiding sex, especially if there has been any bleeding.

The two main areas are structural and chromosomal. The structure can be assessed on ultrasound at around 12–13 weeks, then again in more detail at 19–20 weeks. Either a chorionic villus sample (CVS) or an amniocentesis can confirm whether the chromosomes are normal (see 'Week 11'). A screening test may be used to establish a high-risk population of mothers (see 'Week 12'). A mathematical formula combines your age, ultrasound measurement of the nuchal translucency and a simple blood test for levels of two placental proteins (βhCG and PAPP-A).

MY WEIGHT   51 1/2

MY BELLY WIDTH

APPOINTMENTS   24·02 - Dr Booth   8·45
                  no so nauseas

APPROXIMATELY 213 DAYS TO GO

your baby now measures 3.3 cm (1.3 in) and is becoming mobile. Your baby's proportions are changing. The limbs are growing rapidly, as is the body, so the head doesn't seem as large as it did. The limbs are easily recognisable and move in a coordinated way. Compared to the amount of fluid surrounding it, the baby is quite small, so it has a lot of room in which to move. The yolk sac is no longer adjacent to the fetus and is seen quite separately on ultrasound. It is usually still visible until around 12 weeks' gestation, after which it is absorbed. The cord from the placenta to the fetal umbilical region is also visible.

Diagnosing twins in the first trimester is relatively easy, as is determining if they share one placenta and if they are in the same or different gestation sacs. Identical twins, which tend to share the placenta, are a chance event. The risk of this occurring in different populations is similar. Non-identical twinning is a result of multiple ovulation, which can be more likely if there is a family history, in certain races (for example, African) and as the mother's age increases. Infertility treatment that stimulates the ovaries also tends to cause non-identical twinning.

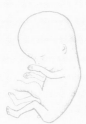

10 WEEK FETUS

SWIMMING

Swimming is recommended during pregnancy as it does not increase the body's temperature as quickly as other sports and the water supports your body's weight.

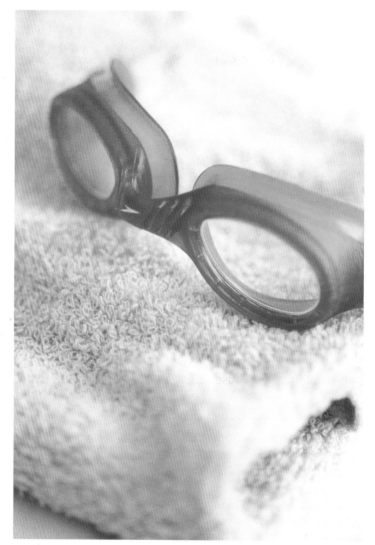

exercise If you had an exercise program before falling pregnant, there is no need to stop. However, during the first trimester tiredness may become an issue, reducing sporting performance. If there has been any bleeding, then it would be best to take it easy until the bleeding has stopped. If your exercise program included impact or contact sports, consult your practitioner. If you've just begun exercising, start slowly and build up your fitness. Always maintain good posture. Sensible exercise during pregnancy includes:

- Walking
- Yoga
- Pilates (a gentle stretching and strengthening form of exercise suitable for pregnant women; it's also very beneficial for back pain)
- Cycling
- Swimming

Exercise at least three times a week. Wear the correct shoes, a sports bra and comfortable clothing. Unless you're swimming, don't exercise in the middle of the day in hot weather. Try first thing in the morning or at the end of the day.

antenatal classes

You can attend antenatal classes from 12 to 40 weeks. It's a good idea to book them early to avoid disappointment. The hospital of your choice may offer them, or you can go to classes run by private organisations. Learn about labour, options for pain relief, what to expect after delivery, common newborn problems, caring for a newborn, babyproofing your house, breastfeeding, bottle-feeding and infant cardiopulmonary resuscitation (CPR). Learning all you can about birth and babies will help you feel more confident, especially if you're a first-time parent.

pelvic floor exercises

Keep up those pelvic floor exercises! The floor of the pelvis is made up of very important muscles which support the organs in the pelvis; these muscles are stretched during pregnancy (see 'Week 31').

Here is one pelvic floor exercise you can do at home or work. Sit forward on a chair with your back straight and your elbows on your knees. Pretend that you are trying to stop passing urine or wind by tightening your pelvic floor muscles. Hold for a few seconds before relaxing completely. Repeat. Start by doing five at a time and build up to as many as you can until the muscles feel tired. You can do a bracket of five several times each day.

YOGA MAT
An exercise or yoga mat is a useful item: use it for relaxation exercises, yoga, Pilates and simple stretching.

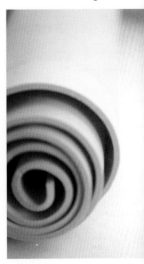

DATE 01·03·09

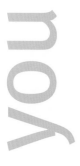

you are nearing the end of the first trimester and may be almost counting down until the nausea ceases, which is usually around week 12 or 13. During this time, while you are still feeling tired and nauseous, decisions about chromosome screening and testing are made. Some women have already made the decision to have a definitive test or, alternatively, not to have any testing, regardless of whether they are considered to be at high or low risk. This could be due to religious beliefs, or possibly the experience of having a disabled relative. Many couples do not have fixed ideas on this topic and may not have given it much thought yet.

Chorionic villus sampling (CVS) involves obtaining a small fragment of placental tissue, which has the same chromosomal make-up as the fetus. Under ultrasound guidance a doctor passes a needle into the placenta. This test can be performed from 11 weeks and involves a small risk of miscarriage. This risk is quite dependent on the skill of the doctor performing the procedure and is in addition to the pre-existing chance of a pregnancy miscarrying anyway.

Amniocentesis is an alternative testing method to CVS. It can be performed from 16 weeks' gestation. A small risk is associated with this test too.

MY WEIGHT   52½

MY BELLY WIDTH

APPOINTMENTS   really tired - a little nauseas

APPROXIMATELY 206 DAYS TO GO

your baby

day by day, the baby grows 1–2 mm (0.04–0.08 in) in length; and by 11 weeks it is 4.4 cm (1.7 in) long. The fetal proportions are continuing to change, with the body and legs growing slightly faster than the head.

The baby is often active but has short sleep–wake cycles, which can be five to 10 minutes long. If the baby is close to waking, a cough can move the baby enough to wake it. Most of the fetal movements are limb movements. There is a small amount of movement of the body and neck, but much less than is seen in the next two weeks. For this reason the CRL measurement is quite accurate at this stage, and becomes progressively less accurate over the next two weeks.

week 12

you

as you approach the end of the first trimester, the nausea and tiredness begin to subside. The hormonal changes occurring are due to the hCG levels declining after their peak in the 11th week.

An ultrasound this week can determine the number of babies, the position of the placenta, the volume of amniotic fluid, the structure of the baby and the size of the nuchal translucency. The nuchal translucency is the measurement of the soft tissue thickness on the back of the baby's neck.

In certain abnormalities, such as Down syndrome, the nuchal translucency tends to be greater. Any problem affecting the way the baby copes with its changing blood volume will tend to cause a larger nuchal translucency. For example, if there were a problem with the structure of the heart, the nuchal translucency would usually be larger.

The nuchal translucency can be combined with the levels of two placental proteins (βhCG and PAPP-A) and the maternal age to give an estimate of the risk of chromosome abnormality specific to that pregnancy. Many couples use the high or low risk classification to help them decide whether to have any further testing such as amniocentesis or CVS.

YOUR NEXT ULTRASOUND

After the 12 week ultrasound, book the next one at around 19 weeks' gestation so you'll get the time slot that suits both you and your partner.

MY WEIGHT _53 1/2_

MY BELLY WIDTH

APPOINTMENTS _10:03 - ultrasound 8:30_
feeling better

APPROXIMATELY 199 DAYS TO GO

your baby

your baby is 5.6 cm (2.2 in) long.

A small nuchal translucency indicates a fetus at lower risk for heart and genetic problems. If the risk determined by the nuchal translucency test is less than 1 in 300 then it is classified as low risk. As 95 per cent of pregnancies are found to be low risk, this screening test will be reassuring for the majority of mothers.

Your baby is as long as... **a matchbox**

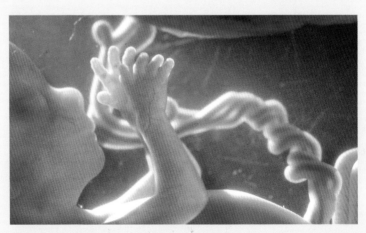

FETUS WITH NORMAL UMBILICAL CORD

when to tell family and friends

Most couples wait until about 12 weeks before sharing their news with friends and family. By this time you will have received the results of blood tests and the nuchal translucency test. The final choice is yours. Tell people when you want them to know.

notes _____

_____

_____

_____

_____

_____

_____

_____

_____

_____

_____

_____

_____

_____

_____

_____

week 13

you

the first trimester has ended. Nausea and tiredness are on the way out but constipation is still relatively common.

By now you are particularly aware of the pregnancy but others around you may not yet notice it. Although you may be able to see all the subtle changes in your appearance, these are not obvious to everyone else. The uterus is not yet large enough to be seen and most of your clothes still fit, although your favourite pair of jeans may not be as comfortable as before.

During most of the first 13 weeks there have been many changes, with some, like tiredness and nausea, being difficult to hide. Keeping these symptoms to yourself while at work can be challenging. Going out and being expected to drink your usual glass of wine can also prove trying. Although ideally you should stick to a regimen of no drugs or alcohol, the occasional glass of wine is unlikely to have any adverse effect. The alteration in your sense of taste may mean that you no longer enjoy the wine so doing without is no hardship. Usually mothers find they have an overwhelming sense of responsibility to protect their unborn babies from anything that may harm them.

MY WEIGHT   54 kg

MY BELLY WIDTH   90 cm (35·5 inch)

APPOINTMENTS   Still got headaches

APPROXIMATELY 192 DAYS TO GO

your baby

your baby now measures 7.0 cm (2.8 in). The heart rate has already started to slow, now beating at 160 beats per minute. Breathing movements can be seen, but of course the fetus is breathing in amniotic fluid. It does not need to breathe oxygen as this is supplied directly by the mother. These breathing movements serve to exercise the chest wall and are essential for lung development.

The kidneys have started to work and the baby's fluid-filled bladder can usually be seen. The amniotic fluid or liquor, which was predominantly fluid that has passed through the skin, changes to being mostly fetal urine. The skin starts to become keratinised, which means that it is more waterproof, stopping the passage of fluid across it.

The placenta is fully formed and has now completely taken over hormone production from the ovaries. Fetal movements are much more complex. Your baby's arms and legs move independently and it can turn its head from side to side.

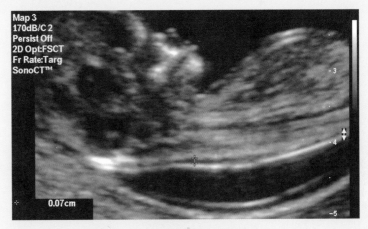

FETUS WITH NORMAL NUCHAL TRANSLUCENCY

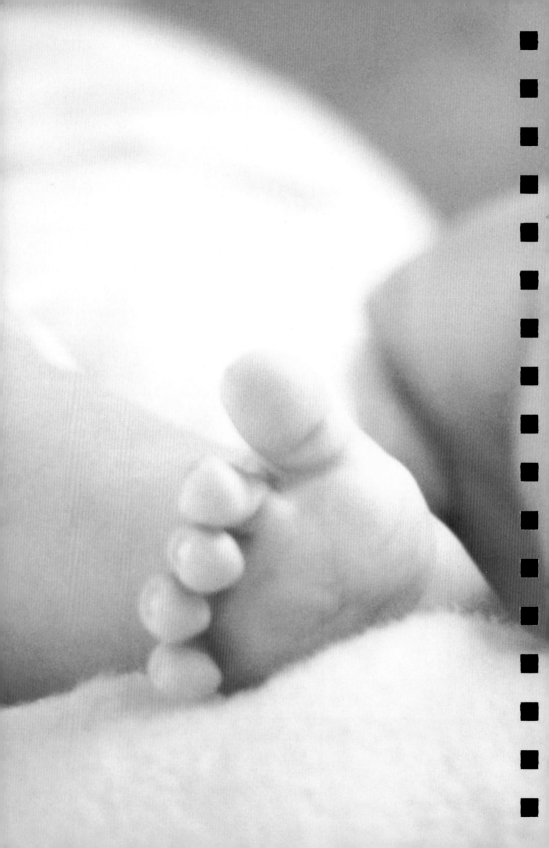

second trimester

you are now entering the 'honeymoon phase' of pregnancy. Chances are your morning sickness is starting to subside, your hair seems thicker and shinier, and your skin is clear, even radiant. In a few weeks you'll be experiencing the flutters of your baby's movements for the first time.

week 14

you

you're officially in your second trimester, the so-called 'honeymoon phase' of pregnancy. That's great news because if your pregnancy has been fairly free of complications till now, your risk of miscarriage is less than 2 per cent. That's a big improvement on the 25 per cent chance of miscarriage that you had at the beginning of your pregnancy. If you have lost a previous pregnancy in the second trimester, it's about this time that your doctor may put a stitch around the cervix to try to make it a little stronger for this pregnancy. This procedure is known as cervical cerclage.

You may be one of the lucky women who find that their morning sickness is subsiding around this time; however, if you're still experiencing nausea, it may continue for a little while longer. Don't worry about this. Your baby is getting all the nourishment it needs, which isn't very much at this stage.

STARTING TO SHOW
You've probably already noticed that your clothes are getting tighter. The top button of your favourite jeans won't do up. Your body is changing.

Your uterus is now a little bigger than the size of your fist, and is growing up from out of your pelvis into your abdominal area. With your bladder empty, you may be able to feel the top of your uterus (called the fundus) about 1 or 2 cm (0.4 or 0.8 in) above your pubic bone in the midline. Don't worry if you can't at this early stage. You will be able to feel it some time in the next few weeks.

MY WEIGHT _54 kg_

MY BELLY WIDTH _91 cm   35·7 inch_

APPOINTMENTS _headaches - mostly sinus_
quesy & constipated

week 14

your baby

the 'alien' you saw at your earlier ultrasound scan is looking far more human, and if you could look inside your womb now, you would see a fully formed baby complete with fingerprints. Your baby measures 7–9 cm (2.7–3.5 in) and weighs 25.5–28.4 g (0.9–1 oz). At this stage, the baby's head and body appear to be more in proportion. Its neck can be clearly recognised, as the head is now up, away from the chest. The eyes have moved closer together and the ears are moving up on the side of the head. Your baby's arms and legs are getting longer, the muscles are beginning to form, and together with the developing joints, allow full body movement. Your baby is moving and jumping hundreds of times a day, secure in its thick-walled uterus, but you would be very lucky to be able to feel it at this early stage.

This is a busy time for your baby. Downy hair, called lanugo, is beginning to grow over its entire body to protect the skin, and will only start to disappear in the few weeks before birth. Head hair and eyebrows are also starting to emerge. The eyelids, fingernails and toenails are beginning to form too. Of course, the eyelids are shut firmly and won't open until about the seventh month of pregnancy. Your baby is starting to produce hormones because its thyroid gland has matured, and about this time the reproductive organs really accelerate in their development. In boys, the prostate gland is now clearly developing, and in girls, the ovaries have begun to descend from high in the abdomen, where they develop close to the kidneys, to enter into the pelvis.

Your baby begins to swallow, the kidneys make urine, and blood begins to form in the bone marrow. During periods of fetal activity, your baby urinates into the amniotic cavity.

DATE **29.03.09**

you

has it sunk in that you're pregnant yet? Many women say that the reality of pregnancy doesn't set in until they trade in their jeans for maternity clothes and others start noticing their swelling abdomen. For many, this realisation is both joyful and scary. It's normal to feel as if you're on an emotional roller coaster (thanks to your hormones).

MY WEIGHT   **55 kg**

MY BELLY WIDTH   **91cm   35.7 inch**

APPOINTMENTS   **03.04.09 -820 - Dr Booth**

APPROXIMATELY 178 DAYS TO GO

your baby

your little baby continues to grow rapidly. It now weighs 49.6 g (1.75 oz) and measures 9–11.5 cm (3.5–4.5 in). It has paper-thin skin through which you can see the network of fine blood vessels coursing over its body. Internally, the bone and marrow in your baby's skeleton continue to develop. The skeleton is getting harder now, transforming from soft cartilage to bone, as the baby continues to lay down calcium. These bones remain flexible, however, so that your baby can pass easily through your pelvis and vagina at birth.

This week the facial muscles become sporadically active and contract to form squints, frowns and grimaces. Your baby isn't upset; its muscles are just contracting involuntarily as part of the normal maturation process. It happens in the arms and legs as well, so your baby's hands will close to form a fist and its feet will point.

Hair growth continues this week on the eyebrows and the head. If your baby is going to have dark hair, the hair follicles may begin to make the pigment that colours the hair. Your baby's ears are almost in position now, although they are still set a bit low on the head.

Sexual development also continues. The genitals are becoming more definite, and it is becoming easier to determine male from female by looking at the external genitalia with ultrasound.

siblings If you are already a parent, it's probably best to wait a little longer than 12 weeks before breaking the news of your pregnancy, especially if your child is a toddler. Explain to your child that there is going to be a new baby brother or sister in the house. Don't ask him whether he would prefer a boy or a girl, as he may be disappointed with the outcome. Include your child in shopping trips for the baby and let him help select clothes or nursery items.

gift for baby Buy a little gift that your child can give to the baby while she is still in hospital. Wrap it and store it in a cupboard, showing him where it is kept (preferably in a high position where he can't reach it, otherwise you may find it unwrapped before the big event!). Tell your partner, babysitter or support person about the gift so it can be taken to the hospital on the first visit.

notes _____

_____

_____

_____

_____

_____

_____

_____

_____

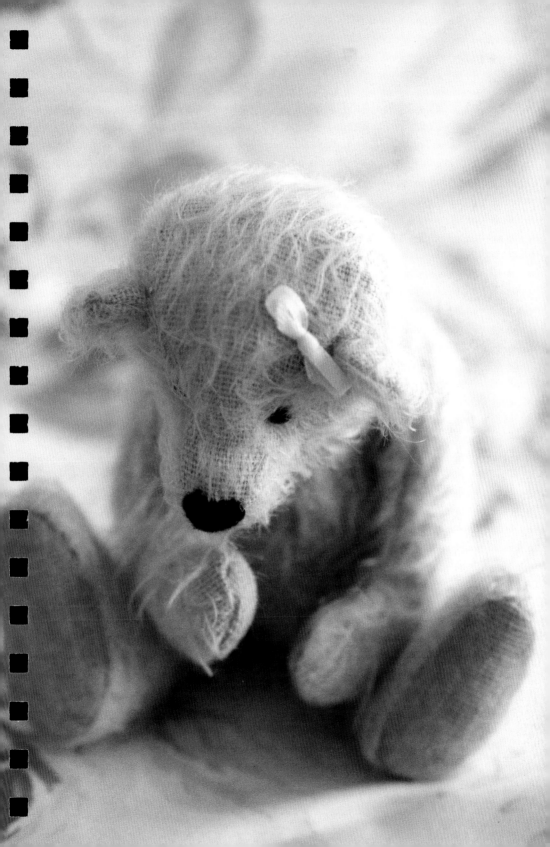

screening tests

It's around this time that you need to consider whether you want to have further tests to determine your risk of having a baby with serious birth defects. There are a few tests done at this stage. If you missed the opportunity to have a nuchal translucency assessment at 11–14 weeks you might want to consider the multiple marker blood screening test for Down syndrome, which goes under many names — the maternal serum screening test, Triple Test, Quadruple Test and Bart's Test, just to name a few. This test is done on a sample of your blood taken between 15 and 20 weeks, and estimates the likelihood of Down syndrome by measuring the levels of alpha-fetoprotein (AFP), a protein produced by the fetus, and the pregnancy hormones hCG and estriol, produced by the placenta.

If the likelihood of Down syndrome is found to be high (that is, greater than a 1 in 250 chance), then you will probably be offered amniocentesis, which will clarify whether your baby does or does not have Down syndrome (or any other chromosomal abnormality) to a very high level of accuracy. Multiple marker blood screening for Down syndrome detects about 65 per cent of pregnancies affected by Down syndrome, which is not as high as the detection rate of the nuchal translucency and first trimester serology screening tests (approximately 90 per cent).

Generally, you are encouraged to have just one of these screening tests, so most women only have multiple marker blood screening in the second trimester if they have missed the opportunity to have nuchal translucency and serology screening in the first trimester.

Another screening test on offer around 15–20 weeks measures levels of AFP in a sample of your blood. The main purpose of this test is to determine your risk of having a baby with serious birth defects such as spina bifida. If you are having

notes _____

_____

_____

_____

multiple marker screening for Down syndrome, measurement of the AFP level is actually included as part of that test. However, it can be requested separately if you do not want or need to have Down syndrome screening at this stage.

In any case, if the test detects an elevated level of AFP in your blood, you will be referred for an expert ultrasound assessment to look for physical abnormalities, particularly spina bifida, that may be affecting the baby. The ultrasound examination is very accurate in detecting those abnormalities associated with a high AFP and, fortunately, where the AFP is raised the majority of babies are found to be normal.

If you're 35 or older, or have a high-risk pregnancy, your doctor may want to discuss amniocentesis with you. Amniocentesis is usually performed around 15–18 weeks and detects chromosomal abnormalities, such as Down syndrome, with 99.9 per cent accuracy. Amniocentesis involves passing a needle into the amniotic sac to sample loose cells from the baby that are floating in the amniotic fluid. These cells are then examined in a laboratory to determine whether the baby's chromosomes are normal. The test also determines the sex of the baby. Amniocentesis is carried out under ultrasound guidance so your specialist can see where the baby is at all times. Despite all the stories in circulation, it is a test that causes minimal discomfort, carrying a less than 0.5 per cent risk of miscarriage when experts do it.

Every couple has different concerns, so talk to your doctor about the pros and cons of having one of the screening tests (multiple marker blood screening for Down syndrome and serum AFP for spina bifida) or diagnostic tests (amniocentesis).

appointments _____

_____

_____

_____

DATE ....

you

you might be starting to feel more energetic around now as you shake off some of the fatigue and anxiety that burdened you earlier in the pregnancy. The nausea should be gone but heartburn may replace it.

The top of your uterus is now out of your pelvis; by the end of this week it will reach to about two to three fingerbreadths above your pubic bone. You will probably find that the pressure on your bladder has decreased because of this, and that you are not going to the toilet as frequently. You can also expect an increase in vaginal secretions if you haven't already. This may be troublesome enough for you to wear a pad.

If you've had babies before, it's about this time that you'll revisit one of the most exciting moments of your pregnancy — feeling your baby move. Unfortunately, your partner won't be able to share in your excitement just yet. Real kicking doesn't usually start for a month or so. If it is your first baby, you may not notice those little flutters and tickles of the baby's activity for a week or two more, especially when you're lying down. Most women notice this 'quickening' between 16 and 20 weeks. Once you realise the baby is doing backflips, note it and tell your doctor or midwife at your next visit.

MY WEIGHT _____

MY BELLY WIDTH _____

APPOINTMENTS _____

APPROXIMATELY 171 DAYS TO GO

your baby is still small enough to fit in the palm of your hand. It measures 10.9–11.7 cm (4.3–4.6 in) and weighs 79.3–85 g (2.8–3 oz). Its skin is transparent and pink in colour. The little hands can grasp and the legs kick actively. The baby's muscles and bones have matured, and its nervous system begins to exert control. Although the first muscle movements were involuntary, this week brings the first voluntary muscle movements. Motion increases as the fetus moves its body and swallows. Your baby can hold its head erect.

What's new this week? Light sensitivity and a bad case of the hiccups, which is a precursor to breathing. You can't hear them, though, because the baby's trachea is filled with fluid rather than air.

Your baby is firmly attached to the placenta via the umbilical cord, which is growing thicker and stronger, thanks to the blood and nutrients constantly rushing through it. The umbilical cord carries nutrients as well as toxins and poisons from tobacco smoke, alcohol and other drugs from the mother to the fetus. The placenta, which nourishes the fetus with nutrients and oxygen and removes wastes, is growing to accommodate your baby. More than 2.5 cm (1 in) thick, it now contains thousands of blood vessels that exchange nutrients and oxygen from your body to your baby's developing body.

If your baby is female, millions of eggs, or ova, form in her ovaries this week.

Your baby is as big as... **an open hand**

week 17

you

break out the elastic-waist pants and maternity clothes. You've probably gained at least 2.2 kg (4.8 lb) by now, perhaps as many as 4.5 kg (9.9 lb). Your uterus is growing and as a result you may feel an occasional pang of pain in the lower abdomen or groin. But it's nothing to be alarmed about — it's just the stretching of your muscles and the ligaments supporting your growing uterus.

As your breasts prepare to nourish your baby after birth, they are changing considerably. The milk lobules and ducts are developing, more blood is flowing to your breasts, and the breast veins become visible, particularly around the nipple and areola (the darkish area around your nipple). Your breasts may have increased by one or two cup sizes, and you may need to buy supportive bras in a variety of sizes to accommodate breast growth during your pregnancy.

At some stage, you and your partner may be feeling a little stressed, worrying about the baby's health, what labour will be like, and how you'll cope as new parents. It's perfectly normal to have these concerns.

MY WEIGHT _____

MY BELLY WIDTH _____

APPOINTMENTS _____

APPROXIMATELY 164 DAYS TO GO

your baby

the baby's movements are becoming stronger and more frequent. Some of your baby's more advanced body systems, including the circulatory system and urinary tract, are working without a hitch now. Your baby has even begun inhaling and exhaling amniotic fluid so its lungs will be strong enough at birth to breathe on their own. It now weighs 99.2 g (3.5 oz) and measures 12 cm (4.7 in).

While most of its organs are in place, your baby is still very thin and lanky. During week 17 your baby starts to form 'brown fat', which will help keep it warm after birth. This type of fat is important in heat production and metabolism. During the last trimester your baby will add other layers of fat to its body for warmth and protection. In fact, in a newborn baby at term, the fat makes up about 2.4 kg (5.3 lb) of its total average weight of 3.5 kg (7.7 lb).

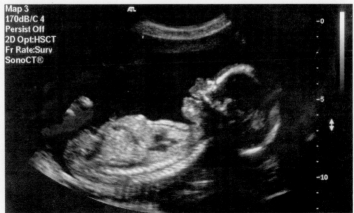

17 WEEKS: THE BABY'S PROFILE, HEART AND SPINE ARE CLEARLY SEEN

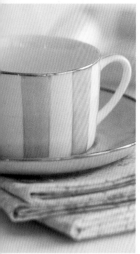

social interaction
While it's nice to talk to your friends about having a baby, you may find that after nine months of pregnancy talk, you'll be fed up, and so will your friends, especially those who don't have children. Try to remember to talk about common interests or local/international issues as well as about the pregnancy. Your own mother may be a great outlet for pregnancy and baby talk. She is unlikely to tire of talking about her imminent grandchild.

emotions
Once the morning sickness stage has passed, some pregnant women feel wonderful. Others feel as if they are on an emotional roller coaster — crying for no reason one minute, feeling ecstatic the next. Go with it, roll with the blows. You're pregnant!

FRIENDS

While most of your friends will be delighted about your pregnancy, a few may be merely disinterested. Try not to feel offended by this.

notes _____

_____

_____

_____

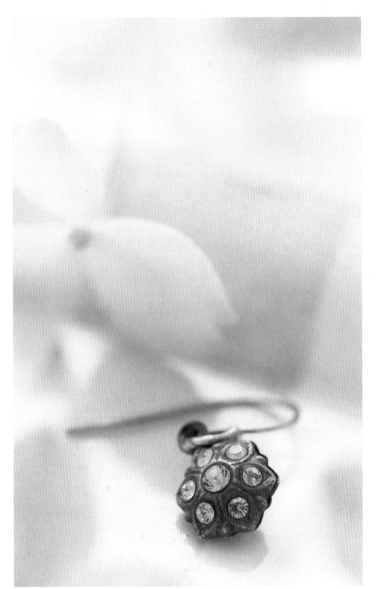

ABSENT-MINDED?

'Maternal amnesia'
is not uncommon
during pregnancy.
You may mislay a
precious item, such
as an earring, or
forget to meet a
friend for coffee.

forgetfulness During pregnancy you will probably find that your memory is not performing as well as it usually does. This could be due to either changes in your hormones and body or just a preoccupation with being pregnant. Many women have been known to go to the supermarket and come home with bags and bags of anything but food! Usually bags full of baby products. This forgetfulness will pass — don't worry about it.

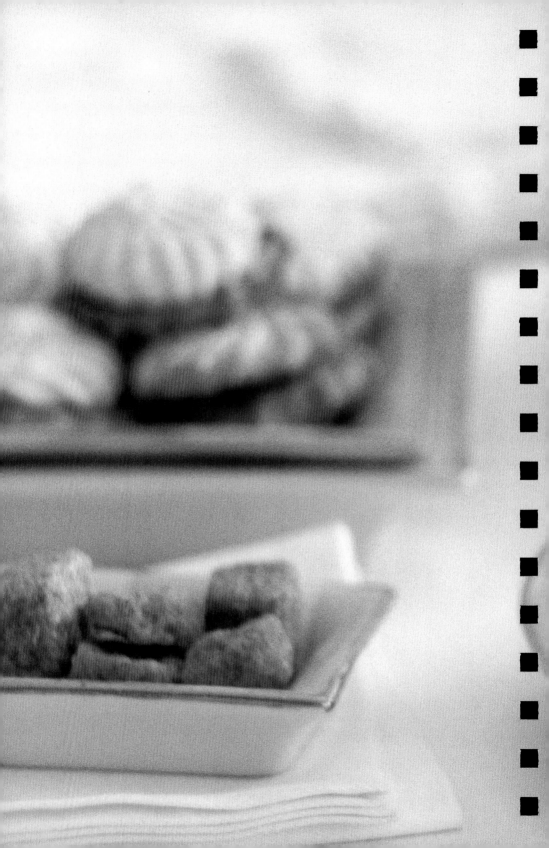

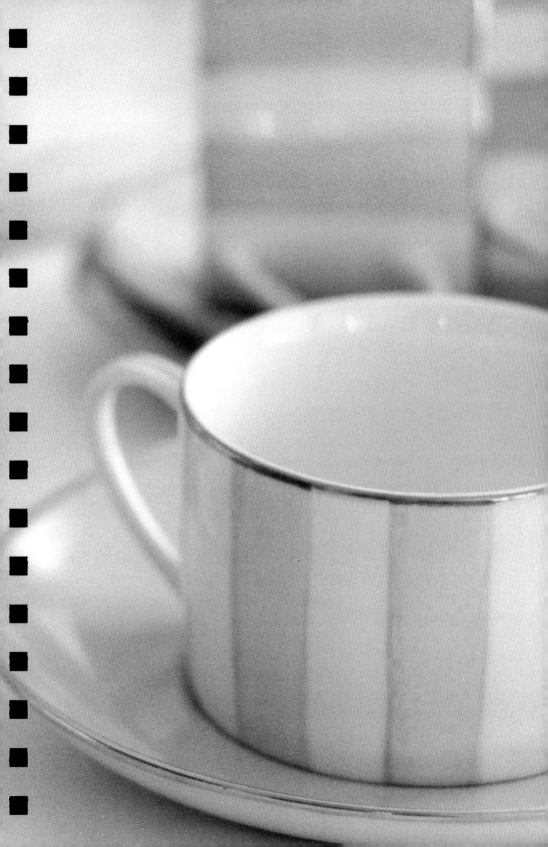

week 18

this week you officially begin your fifth month of pregnancy (that is, you're four months pregnant). The top of your uterus now reaches to halfway between your pubic bone and your navel. If it's your first baby, there's a good chance you'll feel your baby's movements now and in the next few weeks. Many women report that the first sensations are fluttery, or like a butterfly held in the hand. Later in your pregnancy, you'll feel kicks, punches and possibly hiccups!

Your doctor is probably planning for you to have an ultrasound some time between 18 and 20 weeks. If you opt for a mid-pregnancy ultrasound, it will help delineate your baby's anatomy, placental position and fluid volume. While ultrasound can't pick up many of the abnormalities that may be affecting a baby, it is pretty good at picking up physical abnormalities such as spina bifida, cleft lip, kidney disorders and some heart problems. When you see your baby during the ultrasound procedure, you will be amazed at how much it has developed.

Your constant concern for your baby's health may give way to reassurance when everything seems to be okay at your scan. Make sure you take your partner to this exciting examination: you might see your baby kick, flex, reach, roll or even suck its thumb. The sonographer may also be able to determine your baby's sex and will tell you, but only if you want to know.

MY WEIGHT — 55 kg

MY BELLY WIDTH — 93 cm   36·5 inch

APPOINTMENTS

APPROXIMATELY 157 DAYS TO GO

your baby

life is an endless cycle: less than half a year ago your baby was just an egg, but by now, if she's a girl, she has eggs of her own. By now a female fetus's ovaries have already developed the tiny follicles that hold all the eggs she'll ever have — as many as six million, but they will dwindle to one million by the time she's born. Some of her ovarian follicles may even develop and grow, thanks to those female hormones flowing from mother to baby. But these tiny eggs won't develop to the point of ovulation until your daughter reaches puberty.

The baby is continuing to develop, but the very rapid growth rate slows down a little. Your baby looks quite human now. It measures 13–14.5 cm (5.1–5.7 in) and weighs 148.8–155.9 g (5.3–5.5 oz). The unique swirls and whorls that are your baby's fingerprints begin to appear at the tips of its fingers this week. Finite features of the heart — including the chambers, atria and ventricles — are visible during an ultrasound; some abnormalities can be detected. The baby can suck its thumb and has tastebuds.

The bones of the inner ear and the nerve endings from the brain have developed sufficiently for your baby to sense sounds such as your heartbeat and blood moving through the umbilical cord. Your baby may even be startled by loud noises. Its eyes are developing, too: the retinas would probably be able to detect a beam of light if it weren't pitch black in your uterus.

The placenta, that all important nurturing organ, is now almost as big as the baby. Besides providing your baby with a steady diet of nutrients and oxygen, this dark blobby mass also receives waste products from the fetus's blood and deposits them into your bloodstream. Your kidneys then filter out the waste.

week 19

DATE ....

you

welcome to the fifth month of pregnancy. You're just a week away from the halfway mark. Bigger, more comfortable clothes are now a must.

Many women find that their sex drive fluctuates during the various stages of pregnancy. Some find it increases, especially in the second trimester as the nausea goes away and energy returns, but many find it's down. Tiredness, anxieties about the baby, physical changes, work stresses and a host of other concerns have an impact on your libido. Let your partner know how you're feeling. Even though both of you may be preoccupied with the baby, it's important to have some 'together time' too.

You may also be wondering whether having sex will affect your baby. The answer is no. Sex is considered safe at all stages of pregnancy as long as your pregnancy is progressing normally, you haven't had complications in previous pregnancies, and your doctor hasn't suggested you avoid intercourse. Still, you may feel more comfortable just cuddling and 'fooling around' rather than having penetrative sex. Keep the lines of communication with your partner open as these issues come up. You'll probably find he has his own concerns about this also.

MY WEIGHT _____55 kg_____

MY BELLY WIDTH _____

APPOINTMENTS _____

APPROXIMATELY 150 DAYS TO GO

your baby

things are really moving into place now. This week, your baby's eyes look forward instead of to the side, and its ears are in — or nearly in — their final spot on the sides of its head. Your baby now weighs 198.5 g (7 oz) and measures 13.2–15.2 cm (5.2–6 in).

Throughout your baby's body, a fatty substance called myelin is coating and insulating the nerves so that impulses can flow smoothly. The touch of a soft blanket, the sound of your voice — these speedy paths from sensory organs to brain will carry all of these things. Myelination of the spinal cord also takes place.

Over the next few days the buds for the permanent teeth will begin to form behind the milk teeth buds.

The sebaceous glands start producing a greasy white substance called vernix caseosa, a covering that protects the delicate fetal skin from the amniotic fluid. Usually it is largely gone by birth, but babies may still be covered in this cheesy coating if they are born premature.

If you have any
pants that you no
longer wear, cut out
the front section
and sew in a panel
of tracksuit ribbing.
Wear the pants with
a long top or shirt,
and you'll have an
extra item to wear.

pregnancy wardrobe

If this is your first pregnancy, you probably won't need to start wearing maternity clothes until around 16 weeks. Lycra and jersey are fantastic fabrics as they have plenty of stretch. You'll fall in love with elastic waistbands because you'll be too big for your jeans and fitted trousers by about 10 weeks' gestation. Expect to 'pop out' earlier with your second and subsequent pregnancies than you did with your first.

If you plan your wardrobe well, you can keep the expense down. Specialty maternity items can be expensive. You'll probably need larger bras by about 12–14 weeks, as your breasts will have increased in size by then. If you're planning to breastfeed, have yourself fitted for nursing bras at a large department store during your third trimester. Wear bikini briefs as they fit under your tummy.

Basic items

- 2 pairs casual pants
- 1 skirt (at least)
- 4 tops
- 1 cardigan
- 1 swimming costume for summer
- 1 jacket for work, if necessary
- 2 jumpers or sweatshirts for winter
- 1 outfit for going out at night or for more formal occasions

notes _____

_____

_____

_____

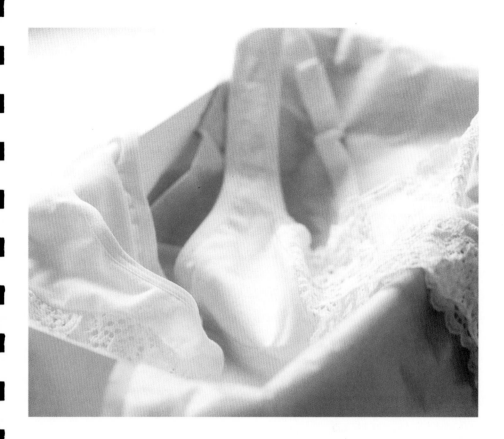

Buy sensibly and always select colours that will match or blend with each other. Try accessorising with scarves, jewellery, hair combs and shoes. Borrow maternity clothes from friends and family.

things to buy

_____

_____

_____

_____

week 20

you

you are halfway through your pregnancy. Your uterus has grown well into your abdomen by this point. By the end of this week the top of your uterus will be about two fingerbreadths below your belly button, or umbilicus. From now on it will grow at a rate of about 1 cm (0.4 in) per week.

You may notice that the areolas of your breasts are getting larger. Each areola can sometimes cover as much as half your breast. It's a harmless side effect of pregnancy that may last as long as 12 months after the birth of your child. Birth is still months away, but your breasts may have already started making the fluid that feeds your baby for the first few days after birth, before your milk starts to flow. Sometimes the nipple may discharge some of this whitish milk, called colostrum, so be prepared with tissues or nipple pads.

You may also be feeling rather scatterbrained. Even the most organised women report that pregnancy somehow makes them forgetful, clumsy and unable to concentrate. Try to keep the stress in your life to a minimum and take your 'mental lapses' in your stride — they're only temporary.

MY WEIGHT   55 kg

MY BELLY WIDTH

APPOINTMENTS

week 20

APPROXIMATELY 143 DAYS TO GO

your baby has grown significantly since it was that first dividing cell. It weighs 255.2–283.5 g (9–10 oz) and measures 14–16 cm (5.5–6.3 in). All its organs and structures have formed, and a period of simple growth begins. By now the baby is so large that its movements are stronger and more easily felt. It is a crucial time for sensory development. The brain is developing specialised areas for the senses — smell, taste, hearing, vision and touch.

Under the covering of vernix caseosa, your baby's skin is thickening and developing layers, including the dermis, epidermis and subcutaneous layer. Hair and nail growth continues this week.

Respiratory movements occur, but the lungs have not developed enough to permit survival outside the uterus.

The fetal heartbeat is growing stronger now. In the latter part of the second trimester, its distinctive 'whoosh-whoosh' can be detected with a simple at-home monitoring device. Your baby's heart beats rapidly — about twice as fast as yours does.

Your baby is as big as... **a banana**

week 21

DATE ....

you

exercise can be a great way to stay in shape during pregnancy and can even keep some symptoms — such as varicose veins, excessive weight gain and backache — at a minimum. But pregnancy is not the time to start training for a marathon; going slowly is the name of the game. Because your ligaments become more relaxed during pregnancy, you're at higher risk for injury, so low- or non-impact exercise — such as yoga, swimming and walking — are preferable. Exercising three to four times a week is fine, but doing more than this may be overdoing it. Talk to your doctor before beginning any exercise program while you're pregnant (see also page 48).

Make sure you're getting enough calcium and iron. Your baby needs calcium to strengthen the skeleton and iron to make red blood cells, among other things. In fact, it's almost impossible to get too much calcium and iron from food alone, as long as you're not overeating. A sensible balanced diet is always best. Iron-rich foods include lean red meat, poultry, fish, lentils, spinach and iron-fortified cereals. Calcium-rich foods include dairy products, but remember, it is advisable to avoid soft cheeses and ricotta. (See also the dietary table on page 26.)

MY WEIGHT   56 kg

MY BELLY WIDTH   95cm   37.5inch   – 13inch 33cm

APPOINTMENTS

APPROXIMATELY 136 DAYS TO GO

your baby is putting on weight but is still only 10 per cent of its final birth weight at this stage. It weighs 297.7 g (10.5 oz) and measures 18.5 cm (7.3 in).

Until now your baby's liver and spleen have been responsible for the production of blood cells. (The fetal liver produces blood cells until the time of birth.) But now the bone marrow spaces are developed enough to contribute to blood cell formation as well.

What does a baby dream about in the womb? This intriguing question arises in the coming weeks as your baby's sleep patterns begin to emerge (although, according to most research, dreaming may not begin until around week 28). When is your baby snoozing? You might be able to tell if its movements show a marked slowdown at certain times of the day. Some scientists suggest that your eating and sleeping habits as well as the levels of light and noise around you function as signals and help your baby set its internal clock to match the outside world's even before birth.

At this point in its development, your baby's brain begins to grow very quickly, especially in what's called the germinal matrix. This structure, deep in the middle of the brain, serves as a kind of factory for brain cells and disappears shortly before birth. But the brain's amazing expansion program continues: its capacity constantly grows until your child reaches the age of five years.

As your pregnancy progresses, meconium begins to accumulate in your baby's bowels. This black goo is the product of cell loss from your baby's bowel loops, digestive secretion and swallowed amniotic fluid. It will appear — usually after birth, although occasionally *in utero* — as baby's first poo.

beauty

Maintaining a good diet and exercise program is the best way to care for your skin, hair and nails during pregnancy. Often a woman's hair and skin look their best during pregnancy.

You may experience some facial discolouration, called chloasma, but this will fade after pregnancy. Sunlight will darken the discolouration. If you are affected by chloasma, make sure you wear a hat and sunscreen when out in the sun.

Your skin may feel dry during pregnancy. Make sure you drink plenty of water and keep applying moisturiser.

On the other hand, your skin may become greasy during pregnancy; pimples may even appear. Use a good quality cleanser, followed by a toner, on your face. Speak with your doctor if the problem disturbs you. If you have a beautician, she may suggest a deep cleansing facial and should give you advice on caring for your skin during pregnancy. This does not mean you will need to purchase a new and expensive range of skin care products. There are very good quality, reasonably priced products available and your skin will return to normal after your baby is born.

If you can afford it, treat yourself to a facial, manicure and pedicure in the last weeks of pregnancy. It will make you feel better and it might be some time before you have the opportunity again. Remember, pregnant women are beautiful.

notes _____

_____

_____

_____

_____

_____

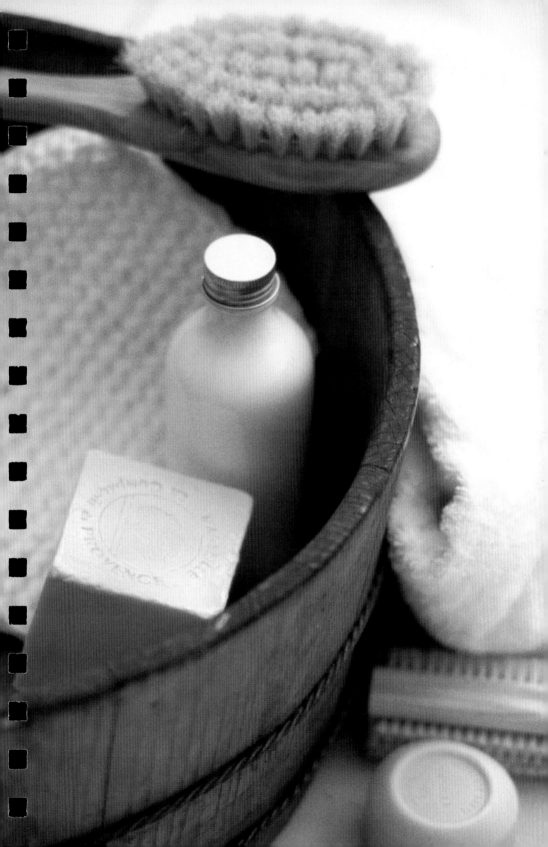

DATE ....

you

it's hard to be a smooth operator when you're pregnant. Don't be surprised if you find yourself being a little clumsy these days. You're carrying more weight, your centre of gravity has changed with your growing uterus, and your hips, fingers, toes and other joints are all loosening due to the effect of pregnancy hormones. Be careful, and if you haven't already, discard your high heels. They make keeping your balance more difficult, and cause backaches. Flat-soled shoes and sandals are more appropriate now.

This week you may begin to notice your uterus having painless contractions called Braxton-Hicks contractions. You may feel a squeezing sensation near the top of your uterus. Don't worry, your baby may be able to feel the contraction as it squeezes the uterus, but Braxton-Hicks contractions aren't dangerous or harmful. It's just the uterus practising for delivery. However, if the contractions become painful or if you have more than four in an hour, contact your doctor: painful, regular contractions may be a sign of preterm labour.

Although pregnancy might sometimes feel like a one-woman show, it doesn't have to be that way. Your partner can help by taking responsibility for researching all the baby equipment you'll need. Stroller, car seat, cot — the list is endless!

MY WEIGHT _____56 Kg_____

MY BELLY WIDTH _____

APPOINTMENTS _____

APPROXIMATELY 129 DAYS TO GO

your baby continues to grow and is getting larger every day. It measures 19.5 cm (7.7 in) and weighs 347.3–368.5 g (12.3–13 oz). Still, there is no real chance that a baby this young could survive outside its mother's body.

Your baby's eyelids and even the eyebrows are developed. The fingernails are visible and cover the fingertips. Organ systems in your baby are becoming specialised for their particular functions. An important function of the liver is the breakdown and handling of bilirubin, a substance produced by red blood cells when they are destroyed. The fetal liver has a limited capacity to convert bilirubin and remove it from the fetal bloodstream. If your baby cannot sufficiently break down this material by birth, it might be slightly jaundiced and need to be placed under lights for a few days.

Sweat glands develop, and the external skin has turned from transparent to opaque. Baby's heartbeat can be heard with a normal stethoscope.

Your baby's reproductive system is continuing to develop, too. In a girl, the uterus and ovaries are in place and the vagina is developed. In a boy, the testes, which have been tucked up inside the pelvis, begin to move towards the scrotum this week. Primitive sperm have already formed in the tiny squiggling passages of the testes. This little boy of yours is already producing testosterone.

notes _____

baby's senses
At this stage the baby has a full range of activity — coughing, hiccups, squinting and even frowning. By the end of this week, your baby's hearing will be well established, thanks to the bones of the inner ear, which have hardened and are able to detect sound vibrations. Your baby can pick up noises from outside the womb and from within — the rush of your bloodstream, the thumping of your heart and even the gurgling of your stomach.

Watch what you say from here on. At birth, your baby will recognise your voice by its frequencies and patterns, so don't be shy about talking to it often during its time *in utero*. Talk, read and sing to your baby. Choose some children's classics or read aloud one of your own books. Some studies suggest that after birth a newborn will suck more vigorously when you breastfeed her if you read to her from a book frequently heard *in utero*. Your partner should chime in, too. In fact, research shows that low-frequency sounds mimicking a male voice penetrate the abdomen and uterine wall better than the higher frequencies of the female voice.

The senses your baby will use to learn about the world are developing daily. Tastebuds have started to function on the tongue, and the brain and nerve endings are formed enough so that the fetus can feel touch. Your baby may experiment with this new-found sense of touch by stroking its face or sucking on a thumb, as well as feeling other body parts and seeing how they move.

week 23

you

at this point, you should be steadily gaining weight — about 0.25 kg (9 oz) each week. You may also notice that your cravings are kicking in. It's okay to give in to an occasional yearning for ice cream, but try to find healthy substitutes if you're longing for junk food.

The closer you are to your delivery date, the more trouble you may have. Anxiety, frequent urination, heartburn, leg cramps and general discomfort can translate into a short night's sleep for a pregnant woman. Try a warm bath, soothing music, a relaxing book or a cup of herbal tea to put you in the mood for sleep. The health of both you and your baby depends on how much rest you have.

Many doctors recommend that pregnant women sleep on their sides, not on their backs or stomachs, so that blood flow to the placenta is not restricted. If you find this position uncomfortable, try placing a pillow between your knees to relieve the pressure of your weight while lying on your side.

MY WEIGHT   57kg

MY BELLY WIDTH

APPOINTMENTS

APPROXIMATELY 122 DAYS TO GO

your baby

by now your baby resembles a small doll with all the facial features of an infant at birth. It weighs 420–520 g (14.8–18.4 oz) and measures 20 cm (7.9 in). Your baby looks like a miniature newborn. The first signs of teeth appear as buds beneath the gum line. Before you know it, your baby will be smiling at you. Your baby's lips are becoming more distinct and its eyes are developed, although the iris (the coloured part of the eye) still lacks pigment. The pigment that colours your baby's skin is being deposited this week. The pancreas is developing; it is very important in the production of insulin, which helps in the utilisation of sugars by the active muscles. Your baby's daily workout routine includes regularly moving the muscles in the fingers, toes, arms and legs. You may feel more forceful movement as a result.

Even though fat is accumulating on your baby's body, the skin hangs loosely, giving your baby a wrinkled appearance. This is due to the fact that the skin is produced more quickly than the fat accumulates.

It's from this point on that your baby may have a chance of surviving outside the womb with expert medical care, but at this age the figures aren't great. If your baby were born prematurely now it would have about a 20 per cent chance of survival but about 50–75 per cent of having some degree of cerebral palsy or other disability.

DATE ....

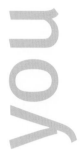

your uterus reaches to just over the top of your umbilicus by the end of the 24th week.

Pregnancy hormones can make your gums sensitive due to increased blood supply, which may result in frequent, easy bleeding, especially when you floss or brush. It's important to practise preventive dental measures during pregnancy in order to avoid decay, so keep brushing and flossing, but gently.

An important prenatal test, the glucose challenge or glucose tolerance test, is usually performed some time during weeks 24–28. This screening test checks for gestational diabetes, a temporary type of diabetes that occurs during pregnancy. Gestational diabetes can cause newborn problems such as low blood sugar. This type of diabetes may also increase the chances of a woman needing a caesarean section because it can lead to the hormonal growth of unusually large babies (macrosomia).

ANTENATAL VISITS
One way your partner can stay involved with your pregnancy is to accompany you to antenatal visits. Not only will he be able to hear first-hand how things are going, he can also have his own questions answered.

During the glucose screening test you'll drink a sugary solution and then have your blood drawn. If your blood sugar levels are abnormal, you'll have further tests, which your doctor will discuss with you. Usually gestational diabetes can be controlled with a strict diet (similar to the one a diabetic follows), but sometimes medication, such as daily insulin, will be needed until the end of the pregnancy.

MY WEIGHT _____ 57 kg _____

MY BELLY WIDTH _____ 15inch   38cm _____

APPOINTMENTS _____

APPROXIMATELY 115 DAYS TO GO

your baby

your baby's eyes can now open as the eyelids begin to separate. Its fingerprints and toe prints are visible. Your baby weighs 570–700 g (1.3–1.5 lb) and measures 21–22 cm (8.3–8.7 in).

The inner ear is now completely developed and controls balance in the body. Your baby may therefore be able to tell when it is upside down or right side up while floating and making movements in the amniotic fluid.

Although your baby is still receiving oxygen via the placenta, once birth occurs its lungs will start taking in oxygen on their own. In preparation for the outside world, airway passages form tubes in order to take in and expel air. Blood vessels and air sacs develop in the lungs; they will eventually exchange oxygen and circulate it to all parts of its body. Your baby's lungs will now begin to produce surfactant. This is a substance that keeps the air sacs in your lungs from collapsing and sticking together when you exhale, allowing you to breathe properly.

All of this means that your baby's lungs have developed enough to increase its chance of surviving outside the womb. Still, a baby born at 24 weeks would have about a 50 per cent chance of survival with intensive care, with about 50 per cent of the surviving babies having disabilities, a third of which would limit quality of life. Clearly, a baby still has a lot of growing to do and ideally will stay put until what is considered full term, at the end of the 37th week.

Your baby is as big as... **a small doll**

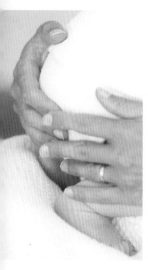

babyproofing

You're probably beginning to prepare for life with baby. However, your preparations should extend beyond gathering the layette and painting the nursery. Your uterus provides a safe haven for your baby before birth. But what about after your baby is born? He or she will be moving about your home in what seems like no time at all. Take the time now, before your baby is mobile, to safeguard your home by babyproofing. Covering electrical outlets, removing choking hazards, installing smoke alarms and blocking off staircases are just a few steps you can take to ensure your child's safety. Take every precaution you can think of, but remember: no amount of babyproofing can substitute for careful supervision of your child.

your toddler

Show your toddler pictures of newborn babies and let him feel the baby moving in your abdomen. Explain as much about the baby as you think he will understand. Tell him that you will be going to hospital for a few days as well as where and with whom he will be staying (if applicable).

notes _____

_____

_____

_____

_____

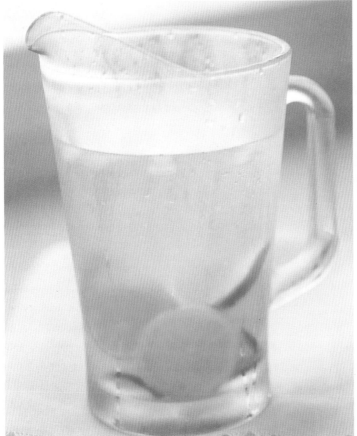

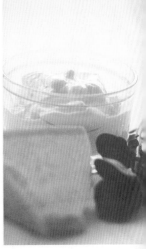

CURE FOR CONSTIPATION
To ease constipation, add oat bran to anything you can think of, such as cereal, yoghurt, smoothies or even pasta sauce.

water is essential Drink it to avoid dehydration, to stop your skin feeling dry and to help prevent constipation, which could lead to hemorrhoids.

notes _____

_____

_____

_____

_____

DATE 07·06·09

you

pregnancy can cause some unpleasant side effects. Your eyes may be sensitive to light and feel gritty and dry. This is a perfectly normal pregnancy symptom called dry-eye. To ease your discomfort, use an artificial tears solution to add moisture.

Not only does the hormone progesterone slow the emptying of the stomach (to allow for increased absorption of nutrients for your baby), but also your expanding uterus is putting increased pressure on your intestines. The result is indigestion and heartburn that can make it difficult to enjoy your favourite meals. Try eating smaller and more frequent meals, and avoid spicy and fatty foods.

If you're going to get stretch marks — and this is genetically ordained — now is about the time they'll show up, on your tummy, breasts, hips or buttocks. These stretch marks are known as stria, and initially look like faint red streaks. Despite manufacturers' promises, creams won't make them go away, but wearing a supportive bra and using moisturiser may help prevent or minimise the stretch marks appearing on your breasts. Stretch marks are typical at this stage of pregnancy and will eventually fade to silvery white marks.

MY WEIGHT — 58 kg

MY BELLY WIDTH — 38cm - 15inch   96cm

APPOINTMENTS — 11·06 at 4:30 - Dr Booth

horrible heart burn this week

APPROXIMATELY 108 DAYS TO GO

your baby

your baby is growing steadily. It now weighs 630–720 g (1.4–1.6 lb) and measures 23 cm (9 in). Its skin is thin and fragile, but its body is filling out proportionally and taking up more room in your uterus. Your baby may also be developing a weakness for sweets. The tastebuds are well formed, and, believe it or not, so is a sweet tooth.

You may notice that your baby has resting and alert periods. Fetal activity is more obvious when you are sitting or lying down.

That crucial lifeline, the umbilical cord, is thick and resilient now. A single vein and two arteries run through it, encased in a firm gelatinous substance called Wharton's Jelly, which prevents kinking and knotting and may regulate the blood flow between placenta and baby. The baby, with its new-found sense of touch, often explores the cord with its hands.

Your baby's permanent 'grown-up' teeth are now developing in buds high inside the gums, but these adult teeth won't come in until the baby teeth (also called primary teeth) start to fall out around the age of six. Meanwhile, nerves around the mouth and lip area are showing more sensitivity now, preparing baby for that all-important task of finding a nipple and sucking for milk. Your baby's swallowing reflexes are developing, too, but at this stage it's only taking in amniotic fluid.

If your baby were born now it would have about a 70 per cent chance of surviving, with only a 20–30 per cent chance of disability, and only a third of these would adversely affect your baby's quality of life.

DATE ....

you

your uterus now reaches to one or two finger-breadths above the level of your navel.

Sleep may not feel that restful any more, and you may be having vivid and scary dreams. When you sleep, your subconscious becomes a staging area for your fears and insecurities about pregnancy and impending motherhood. Your baby's activity is reassuring but sometimes a lack of activity may worry you. Each baby has different movement patterns, but if you are concerned about your baby's movement, or if you feel the movements have decreased in frequency or intensity, talk to your doctor.

If your doctor previously screened you for pregnancy anemia (a deficiency of red blood cells), you may be screened again around this time. Many pregnant women develop a mild anemia because of normal changes in their bodies.

MY WEIGHT _____

MY BELLY WIDTH _____

APPOINTMENTS _____

week 26

your baby still looks wrinkly, but it will continue to gain weight steadily over the next 14 weeks until birth. Its weight — 680–750 g (1.5–1.7 lb) — is now about 25 per cent of its expected term birth weight. Three-quarters of its weight will be put on in the last 14 weeks! To support the fetus's growing body, the spine is getting stronger and more supple. Although no longer than the span of the average adult hand, it is now made up of 150 joints and some 1000 ligaments. Your baby now measures 25 cm (10 in).

The baby can now inhale, exhale and even cry. Fetal brain scans at 26 weeks show that your baby now responds to touch. Also, if you shine a light on your abdomen, your baby will turn its head, which researchers say shows some functioning of the retina and optic nerve.

Depending on racial background, some babies will be born with blue or grey-blue eyes (which may change colour in the first six months of life) and some will be born with brown or dark eyes. Eyelashes are growing in, as is more hair on the head.

Feel like your baby is bouncing off the walls? It's no wonder — baby's living quarters are getting pretty snug these days. If you're lucky, your partner will not only be able to feel movements, but will also be able to detect the baby's heartbeat when his ear is pressed against your uterus.

If your baby were born now it would have about an 80 per cent chance of surviving, with only a 20–30 per cent chance of disability, and only a third of these would adversely affect quality of life.

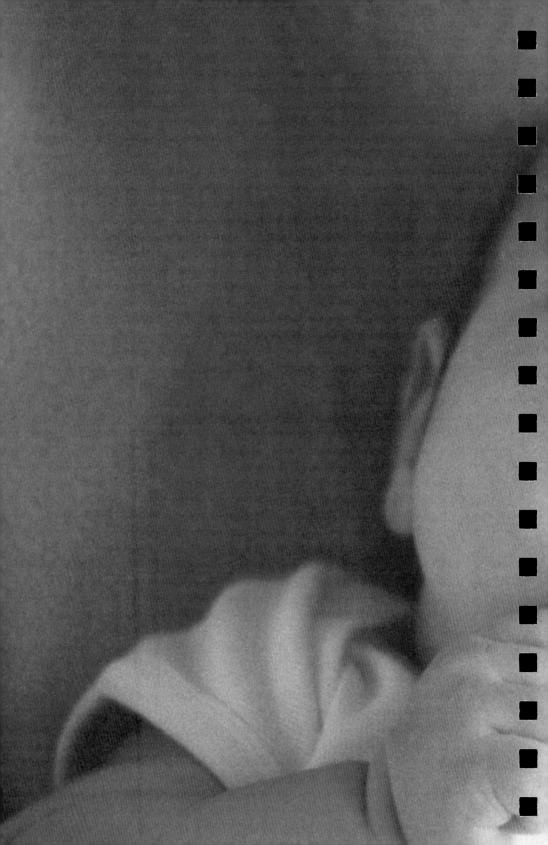

third trimester

you are now entering the last trimester, which means that you are two-thirds of the way through your pregnancy and literally entering the home straight.

week 27

you

your fundus should now be almost halfway between the umbilicus and the bottom of the ribcage (xiphisternum), and disorders such as heartburn are becoming more prominent. You can try easing this problem by sleeping propped up on a few pillows, although this may not be the most comfortable position for sleeping.

In fact, as your pregnancy advances, you will find it increasingly difficult to get into a comfortable sleeping position. When lying on your side, use extra pillows under your stomach and between your knees. When on your back, put them under your knees and neck. You'll also probably be up through the night to empty your bladder. If sleeping becomes a problem, talk to your doctor.

Pressure symptoms are becoming more prevalent with possible varicose veins as well as ankle swelling (oedema). You can relieve this by wearing support stockings. For maximum benefit, fit the stockings on before getting out of bed in the morning. They may not look glamorous but should prevent unnecessary discomfort and disfigurement. Other helpful measures include putting your feet up when you can; avoiding prolonged standing, excessive weight gain and tight clothing; and regularly doing some moderate exercise, such as walking for 20 minutes a day.

SWOLLEN FEET
Wrap swollen feet in a cold wet cloth, elevate them and sit under a fan to cool.

MY WEIGHT   59

MY BELLY WIDTH

APPOINTMENTS

THIRD TRIMESTER

your baby

the baby now measures around 30 cm (12 in) and weighs about 1 kg (2.2 lb). If it were to be delivered now it is more likely to survive than not, although there is still a chance of handicap because of the degree of prematurity. This is largely due to breathing problems but prematurity can result in other serious disability, so it is best for your baby to remain in the womb until at least 32 weeks, when the chance of intact survival is far greater.

The placenta is now virtually fully developed, and you are about to embark on the maximum fetal growth phase where baby not only lengthens but also fills out significantly by developing subcutaneous fat. The baby's movements are more tumultuous but a definite rest–activity cycle is now also developing. This becomes more pronounced as full term approaches.

If your pregnancy is complicated by high blood pressure (hypertension), diabetes or twins, or if there is a history of small babies (growth retardation), your obstetrician may suggest a further ultrasound to assess fetal growth and wellbeing over the next few weeks. This may be repeated regularly if there is concern about ongoing development. In general, babies of hypertensive mothers tend to be smaller than average and those of diabetic mothers tend to be larger. At birth these latter babies may be hypoglycemic — that is, have low sugar levels — as they have high levels of insulin, which is what makes them grow excessively. They will need to be fed quickly and kept warm. They are not born diabetic, however.

DATE ....

you may have some more blood tests at this time to assess your blood count, as well as a further antibody screen if you are Rhesus negative, and a screen for diabetes (short glucose tolerance test). A vaginal swab is also often done at this time to exclude beta hemolytic streptococcus infection. These bacteria often colonise the cervix and although this infection is usually not associated with any symptoms, it can cause severe neonatal infection in the baby. It is best to treat it before, rather than after, vaginal delivery.

MY WEIGHT   <u>60 kg</u>

MY BELLY WIDTH

APPOINTMENTS

APPROXIMATELY 87 DAYS TO GO

your baby

the baby has its own regular cycle of quiet and active sleep, and may open and close its eyes as well as suck its thumb. It now measures around 34 cm (13 in) and weighs about 1.2 kg (2.6 lb). Its body is thin and its skin is covered with fine hair-like lanugo as well as a protective layer of the creamy, waxy substance called vernix caseosa.

The placental blood flow is increasing dramatically to accommodate maximal fetal growth over the next eight weeks. This usually tapers off towards the end of pregnancy.

Your baby is as large as... **a football**

week 29

you

as the birth approaches you will be feeling a combination of excitement and exhaustion. Your uterus is getting bigger and heavier, and breathing and sleeping may become more difficult. Not only does the baby weigh well over 1 kg (2.2 lb), but there is also the placenta and around 1 L (1.8 pt) of amniotic fluid present, so it's no wonder you're experiencing some discomfort. Sleeping on your side may help, and extra pillows can help support you in a more comfortable position. The shortness of breath is also due to the growing uterus pushing up on your diaphragm, thus reducing your lung capacity. You compensate for this by breathing more deeply but the sensation of more laboured breathing remains.

MY WEIGHT _____60_____

MY BELLY WIDTH _____

APPOINTMENTS _____

THIRD TRIMESTER

week 29

your baby

if the development of the placenta has been suboptimal, this growth phase may not be as dramatic and may indeed stall completely. Diseases such as hypertension and diabetes may affect placental development adversely, and fetal disorders such as Down syndrome may also limit fetal growth. Measuring umbilical artery blood flow using Doppler ultrasound techniques can indirectly assess placental function. This may allow your doctor to predict whether your pregnancy is at risk of intra-uterine growth retardation.

Your baby weighs 1.5 kg (3.5 lb) and measures 36 cm (14 in).

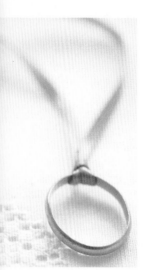

old wives' tales

You will hear some fascinating old wives' tales relating to the symptoms you are experiencing in pregnancy. For instance, heartburn is supposed to be a sign of the baby's hair growing, and if your tummy protrudes more to the front, the baby will be a girl.

It's best to accept the well intentioned advice with a smile. You'll receive many more snippets of wisdom once your baby is born, and while some of these wives' tales have no scientific basis, they have been passed down over many generations by women caring for their babies. Keep an open mind. You'll discover that some of them are true, no matter how unscientific they seem!

BOY OR GIRL?
Another old wives' tale: swing your wedding ring on a piece of ribbon over your pregnant belly. If it goes around in a circle it's a boy, if it swings back and forth it's a girl.

choosing a support person

As labour usually takes some hours, having a support person present, if only to have someone to talk to between contractions in the early stages of labour, is invaluable. Once labour is established, you'll appreciate someone being there to support and encourage you.

Witnessing the birth of a child is the most beautiful experience a couple can share. It will create strong and lasting bonds for mother, father and baby. You'll probably want the baby's father to be your main support person, but you may ask someone else to be present as well — your sister, mother or a particularly supportive, caring friend.

Going it alone

Due to changing circumstances or by choice, some women go through pregnancy without a partner. If you are single and pregnant, choose a calm and caring support person who loves you — your mother, your sister or a friend. You will want to share the changes you are experiencing in pregnancy with someone. It's only natural!

choosing a name for baby

Parents usually take months to choose a name for their baby. They may settle on a name, only to change it a week later. This can go on for several months, even until after the birth. Generally, couples select a name they both like. Some follow tradition and choose family names. If you have other children already, include them in the selection process. It's nice for a young child to think he picked his little brother or sister's name.

week 30

you

in the third trimester your antenatal visits increase from monthly to every second week until 36 weeks. Beyond this stage you should be seeing your doctor or midwife weekly so that she can monitor your progress. During these visits your weight is checked. By this time you should be gaining around 0.5 kg (1.1 lb) per week. Excessive weight gain may be a sign of fluid retention and developing hypertensive disease of pregnancy or diabetes. Inadequate weight gain may indicate intra-uterine growth retardation.

Your doctor or midwife will also check your blood pressure, as well as a urine sample for sugar and protein. She will palpate your abdomen to check the baby's size and position, and will also check the baby's heartbeat by listening to it through a special stethoscope shaped like a trumpet. Finally, she will check your hands, feet and ankles for swelling (oedema).

MY WEIGHT _____

MY BELLY WIDTH _____

APPOINTMENTS _____

week 30

your baby

the baby now measures 37.5 cm (15 in) and weighs around 1.6 kg (3.8 lb). The lungs and digestive system are approaching maturity and from now on your baby's weight gain will exceed its growth in length.

The brain starts to take on a wrinkled appearance because of its rapid growth. This is normal and necessary as this convoluted structure allows for an increased number of brain cells, making your baby's brain capable of integrating the high level of neurological function that will be required for normal life.

During the next month your baby will actively absorb and start to store nutrients that your body provides. This includes calcium for skeletal development, iron for red blood cell production and protein for general growth.

DATE ....

you

this is a good time to start considering your birth plan. Naturally you want everything to go smoothly, from the time labour commences until delivery. A birth plan can facilitate this process and make this special time more meaningful and memorable. A birth plan is an informal agreement between you, your partner, your doctor and/or your midwife about such issues as your preferences for anesthetic, whom you want present at the birth and whether or not you wish to breastfeed. It is important to ask your doctor or midwife if he or she will abide by such a plan, provided all goes well and your birth is a normal, uncomplicated vaginal delivery.

Don't forget to do your pelvic floor exercises at this stage, as with increasing pressure on your bladder, stress incontinence (slight leaking of urine when you cough or laugh) is likely to occur. To prevent ongoing problems after the birth, regularly exercise to strengthen your pelvic floor muscles. These are the broad, flat muscles that attach to the bony pelvis laterally and to each other where they meet in the midline, but are incomplete where the urethra, vagina and rectum pass through them. They support everything above them in humans because they stand erect. If they are weak they are more likely to allow organs above to 'prolapse'.

MY WEIGHT _____

MY BELLY WIDTH _____

APPOINTMENTS _____

APPROXIMATELY 66 DAYS TO GO

your baby

since the baby's eyelids are now unfused, they can open and close. Your baby's eye movements become increasingly obvious in anticipation of birth.

Your baby now weighs 2 kg (4.4 lb) and measures 39 cm (15 in).

DATE ....

you

from around 20 weeks you will probably have noticed painless contractions, called Braxton-Hicks contractions. These become much more intense in the third trimester and may become more frequent. As you are no doubt anxious to know when 'true' labour is starting, it is important to differentiate between the two.

As Braxton-Hicks contractions do not lead to cervical shortening and dilation they are not a sign of true labour. They are usually not painful, and stop when you get up and move around. There is also no 'show' (passing of the mucous plug from the cervix which is usually slightly bloodstained) associated with 'false' labour. But if you are uncertain, a quick visit to the hospital or your doctor can usually resolve this. Many women will have a practice run such as this and it may not be such a bad thing to familiarise yourself with the procedures involved.

MY WEIGHT _____

MY BELLY WIDTH _____

APPOINTMENTS _____

APPROXIMATELY 59 DAYS TO GO

your baby

the baby now measures approximately 40 cm (16 in) and weighs around 2.2 kg (4.9 lb). The skin is still reddish but rather wrinkled, with some early fat deposits. The bones of the head remain soft and flexible, and the lungs have developed to the extent that they can support life. If born now, the baby will almost certainly survive unless it is severely compromised. It can probably hear loud noises and feel some touch, responding with increased fetal movements.

There is also a noticeable reduction in the amplitude of fetal movements as the baby starts to run out of room. It still sleeps 90–95 per cent of the time, but a variation between day and night is becoming more obvious with increased movements at around 3 to 5 am when you are at rest. This may be due to reduced steroid levels in your circulation in the early hours of the morning and is completely normal, although it may disrupt your sleep. It may be inadvertently preparing you for that early feed after the birth.

Your baby is as large as... **a small baguette**

DATE ....

you

you may be developing some stretch marks on your abdomen by now, if you haven't already. These are red or pink striations that may appear on the abdomen, hips and even breasts. Although they will become pale and less obvious after the birth, there are some things that you can do to try to reduce them. First, try not to gain excessive weight as weight gain in a short period of time makes them worse. Rubbing skin softeners into the skin can also help to nourish the skin and keep it supple. If all else fails, rest assured that they will fade over time (see also 'Week 25').

MY WEIGHT

MY BELLY WIDTH

APPOINTMENTS

week 33

your baby

the baby now measures around 41 cm (16 in) and weighs about 2.3 kg (5.7 lb). Your fundus is just below the ribcage and the fetal head is often above the pelvis, where it usually ends up, as there is generally more room there than in the fundus. This is because there are bony margins to the pelvis, and the fundus is muscular and competing with the bowel and liver for space. If your placenta was low lying at your 18–20 week scan, it may be a placenta previa (placenta entering the lower uterine segment), which may prevent the fetal head from entering the pelvis. You may have another ultrasound examination at this time to exclude this possibility.

It is also possible to assess fetal growth and wellbeing at this stage by performing ultrasound measurements on the baby as well as assessing the amount of amniotic fluid present and observing fetal behaviour. This includes fetal movement, tone and breathing, as well as possibly a fetal heart rate trace (cardiotochograph, or CTG). Fetal breathing is of course not real breathing, as the placenta is providing oxygen as well as nutrition at this stage, but 'practice breathing', where baby inhales amniotic fluid. Episodes of fetal breathing become longer and more frequent towards the end of pregnancy and are a sign of fetal wellbeing. Placental and fetal blood flow can also be assessed using Doppler ultrasound.

DATE ....

you

from now on, it may no longer be sensible to travel long distances from home, particularly not by aircraft, as labour may start at any time and you don't want to be miles away from your doctor or hospital. If you feel you must travel, it is important to consult your doctor, and if you must travel by air, she may need to give you a note to say that it is still safe for you to do so. Otherwise the airline personnel may not let you board the aircraft (for details see page 123).

MY WEIGHT   _____

MY BELLY WIDTH   _____

APPOINTMENTS   _____

your baby

some doctors routinely organise a scan at this time to assess the size and condition of the fetus. When there is a risk of growth retardation or fetal compromise due to maternal illnesses, such as diabetes or hypertension, your doctor may perform this scan every second week and even more frequently towards term. As there are still no known detrimental effects of ultrasound examination on the baby this is considered perfectly safe; however, this technology should only be used when clinically indicated.

Your baby weighs 2.3 kg (5 lb) and measures 42 cm (16.5 in).

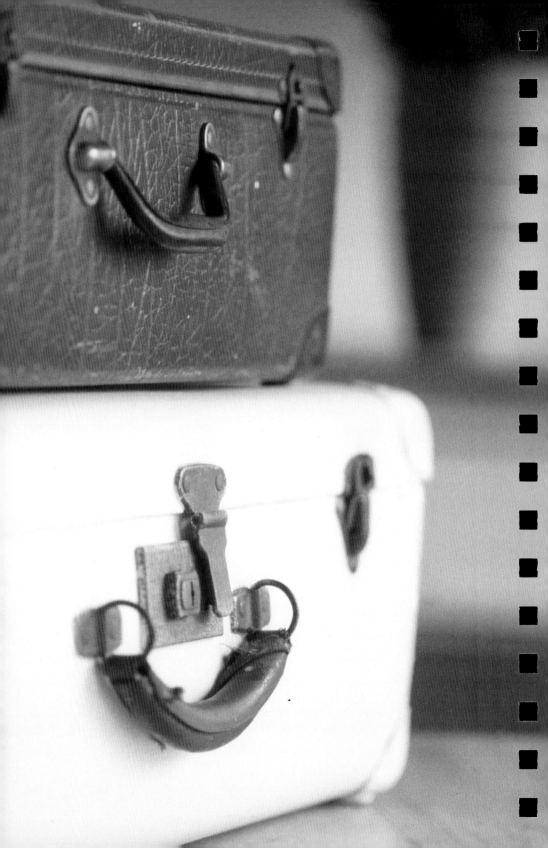

air travel Domestic airlines generally allow you to travel up until 36 weeks as long as you haven't had any complications during your pregnancy; you will be able to travel on international flights up until 34 weeks.

Speak with your doctor before you fly and check airline policies relating to pregnant passengers. Ask for an aisle seat so you can move around the cabin to avoid deep vein thrombosis, and go to the toilet without having to climb over other passengers. A big tummy and economy class seating will make this impossible! Remember to drink plenty of water during long flights.

notes _____

_____

_____

_____

_____

_____

_____

_____

_____

_____

_____

DATE ....

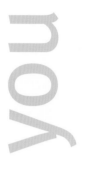

your uterus has now reached the bottom of your ribcage and may cause some discomfort. You may find it more difficult to maintain your balance and that you have to throw your shoulders back in order to counter the weight of your uterus. Your ankles are likely to swell (although you will have difficulty seeing them). You are starting to feel more and more like a 'beached whale'. It is also becoming increasingly difficult to find a comfortable position for sleep. As fetal activity is also most prominent in the early hours of the morning and your baby's vigour is increasing, despite ever diminishing room, you may awake with a start following a swift kick to the gall bladder.

This is also the time of your final blood tests — a full blood count to exclude anemia as well as a repeat antibody test if you are Rhesus negative.

MY WEIGHT _____

MY BELLY WIDTH _____

APPOINTMENTS _____

APPROXIMATELY 38 DAYS TO GO

your baby

fetal behaviour is becoming more structured, with definite rest activity cycles alternating with defined episodes of increased movement that last up to 20 minutes.

This week your baby weighs 2.4 kg (5.3 lb) and measures 44 cm (17 in).

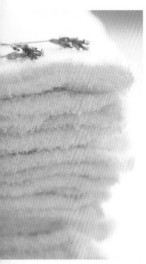

preparing the nursery

For most parents, decorating and preparing the nursery for their first baby is an exciting and fulfilling aspect of pregnancy. Here's a list of basic requirements.

Bassinet/cot

If you're buying a second-hand cot or bassinet, particularly if it is antique or old, make sure the original paint does not contain lead. (Lead poisoning in children can lead to learning disabilities, reduced IQ, impaired hearing, kidney and central nervous system damage, even death.) If you are restoring or painting the cot, check with your hardware supplier that the paint or lacquer you are using is suitable. It is wise to buy a new, good quality mattress and ensure that the cot or bassinet conforms with the relevant standards. Make sure the lock is secure and cannot be opened by a child. Also check that no part of the cot or lock can trap little fingers. To avoid the possibility of suffocation, do not use pillows or cot bumpers.

You'll need three sets of bassinet/cot linen (sheets), preferably in 100 per cent cotton, and three blankets.

Change table

Take the time to choose this very important item carefully. Go for one with lots of pockets or shelves which can hold all the items you'll need at change time — nappy wipes, nappy cream, nappy liners, spare pins and soft toys to amuse baby during changes. Make sure the table is strong and stable, and that it has a restraining belt and high sides so baby can't roll off. Finally, ensure that it is the right height for you: if you have to bend over to change baby, your back will suffer.

SPRING-CLEAN

Ask your partner to help you give the house a thorough spring-clean before your baby's birth.

Never leave your baby on a change table. If you need to reach for something or turn away, keep one hand on your baby. If you need to leave the room, take baby with you or place her in her cot.

Baby needs

- 3 dozen cloth nappies
- 1 pack of disposable nappies
- Nappy liners
- Nappy bucket and a nappy-soaking solution
- Baby wipes

Other useful items in the nursery

- Lamp
- Nappy stacker
- Baby wraps (cotton, cheesecloth or muslin) for settling baby
- Mobile
- Bouncinette or rocker
- Music
- Nursery monitor
- Brightly coloured pictures on the walls
- Chest of drawers
- Wardrobe
- Soft toys
- Rattles

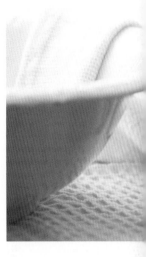

baby's bathtime For baby's bathtime you'll need the following items.

- Baby bath
- 2 face washers
- 2 towels
- Baby liquid soap/shampoo
- Cotton buds
- Cotton wool balls
- Nappy lotion/cream

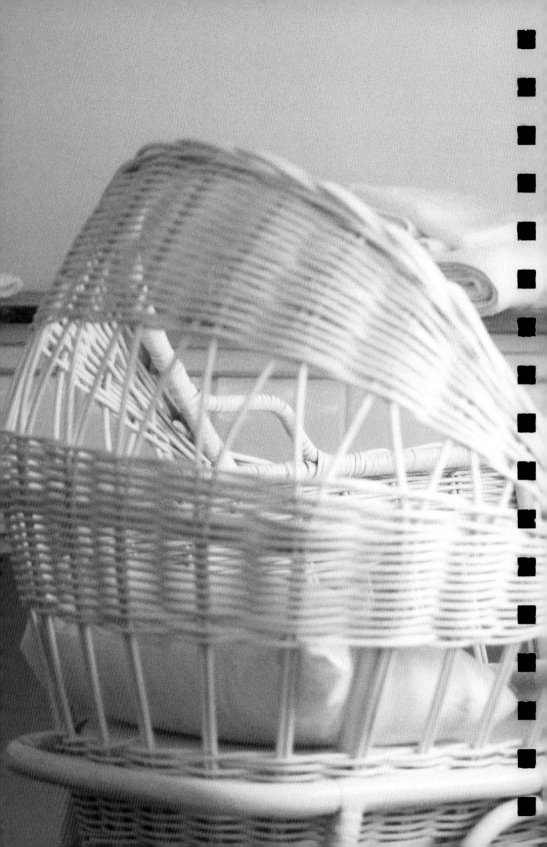

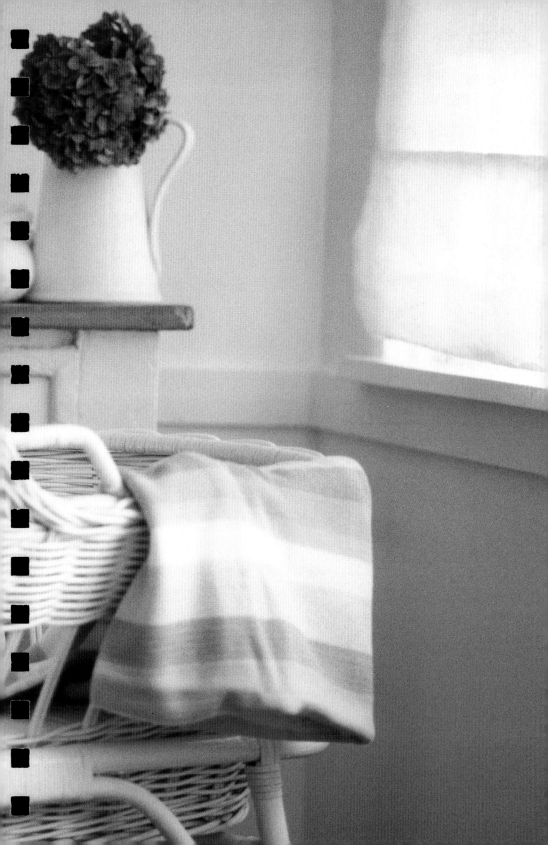

DATE . . . .

you

most expectant mothers who have been working up to this point finally give up. But it is a busy time at home: the baby could literally come at any time and there are still many things to be done. This domestic activity is generally termed 'nesting' and is most pronounced in the first pregnancy. You may feel that you need to clean and reorganise everything.

It is a magical time in many ways, particularly if you have just left the workforce for the first time in order to set up a home for your new family (see 'Preparing the nursery' on page 126). This activity will probably generate an escalating sense of excitement as the concept of motherhood rapidly becomes a reality.

Your partner will also share this excitement but not perhaps with the same sense of fear. Although your relationship is likely to grow closer during this time, it may become less physical: sexual activity may become less comfortable and even rather scary. 'What if we hurt the baby?' is a common concern. Fortunately, this is highly unlikely, although you may need to modify your technique to avoid penetration.

Although you may be feeling increasingly unattractive as your pregnancy progresses, the converse is often true. At this stage of pregnancy you may be particularly radiant. Your altered body contours may be uniquely appealing to your partner.

MY WEIGHT _____

MY BELLY WIDTH _____

APPOINTMENTS _____

week 36

APPROXIMATELY 31 DAYS TO GO

by 36 weeks the baby measures approximately 46 cm (18 in) and weighs about 2.5 kg (5.5 lb). Its hearing is now mature and it is approaching the end of the maximum growth phase. The amount of subcutaneous fat is increasing, giving the baby a more rotund appearance, especially around the face and shoulders, rather than the previous wrinkled look. The fingernails now reach the end of the fingers. If born now the baby will have well over a 90 per cent chance of intact survival.

Your baby is as long as... **a rolled newspaper**

DATE ....

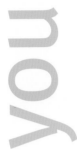

this is the time you should start to pack your bag for that inevitable trip to the hospital or birth centre. Include any special things that you may need in labour, plus items required for your postnatal stay (see 'Packing your bag for hospital' on page 134).

With your progressively reduced tolerance for exercise and increasing difficulty sleeping at night, an afternoon nap is also becoming essential. This is a good habit to develop as you will be feeding during the night in the near future and an afternoon catch-up nap will help you to cope with the inevitable sleep deprivation. Increasing rest with your feet up also helps reduce ankle swelling and discomfort.

COOK EXTRA QUANTITIES
During the last few weeks of your pregnancy, whenever you cook dinner, cook double the quantity and freeze the rest. You'll have a supply of quick meals once you're back home with your new baby.

MY WEIGHT _____

MY BELLY WIDTH _____

APPOINTMENTS _____

APPROXIMATELY 24 DAYS TO GO

your baby

your baby now measures around 48 cm (19 in) and weighs around 2.8 kg (6.3 lb). Fetal movement is now beginning to diminish because conditions in the womb are becoming increasingly cramped. However, as long as you can feel the baby wiggle or bump during the day, every day, you can feel secure in the knowledge that it remains healthy and strong.

full petrol tank Towards the end of your pregnancy, make sure the petrol in the car never gets below half full. You may have to make a dash to hospital at 2 o'clock in the morning.

calling an ambulance If you are alone at home and the onset of your labour is very rapid, you will need to call an ambulance. Give clear directions over the phone if your house is difficult to find. Unlock your front door to enable the paramedics to gain entry when they arrive. If it's night-time, turn on both the interior and exterior lights.

packing your bag for hospital Pack your bag for hospital about four weeks before your due date, just in case the baby surprises you with an early arrival. Pack a smaller bag with the items you'll need when you're in labour and put it inside your suitcase. Use the lists opposite as a packing guide.

notes _____

_____

_____

_____

_____

_____

_____

_____

_____

Labour

- Toiletries bag – face washer, soap, moisturiser, head band or elastic (for longer hair)
- Dressing gown and slippers
- Nightgown or large t-shirt
- Pair of socks (in case of cold feet)
- Massage oil or cream
- Personal tape or CD player plus a choice of relaxing music
- Lip moisturiser
- Camera (remember to ask hospital staff if it's all right to take photos or video the event)
- List of names and telephone numbers of people you will want to call from hospital
- Books or magazines for you and your partner
- Snack foods and drinks for your partner

Hospital stay

- Toiletries and make-up
- Tissues
- 3 nursing bras (although the trend these days is to wear crop tops or t-shirts in hospital)
- Large exercise/crop tops or t-shirts, loose button-through shirts
- Elasticised pants or track pants
- Nighties or pyjamas (preferably with a front opening for breastfeeding)
- Dressing gown
- Slippers
- Underpants
- Breast pads
- 2 packets of maternity pads or large, absorbent sanitary pads
- Small amount of cash for newspapers and telephone calls
- Books and/or magazines
- Pen and paper
- Watch
- Snack foods such as dried fruit or nuts
- Pair of baby mittens as some babies tend to scratch themselves
- Clothes for going home and/or going out
- Set of baby clothes for baby to wear home, including singlet, nappy and pilchers, stretch suit, booties, shawl and bonnet if it's cold

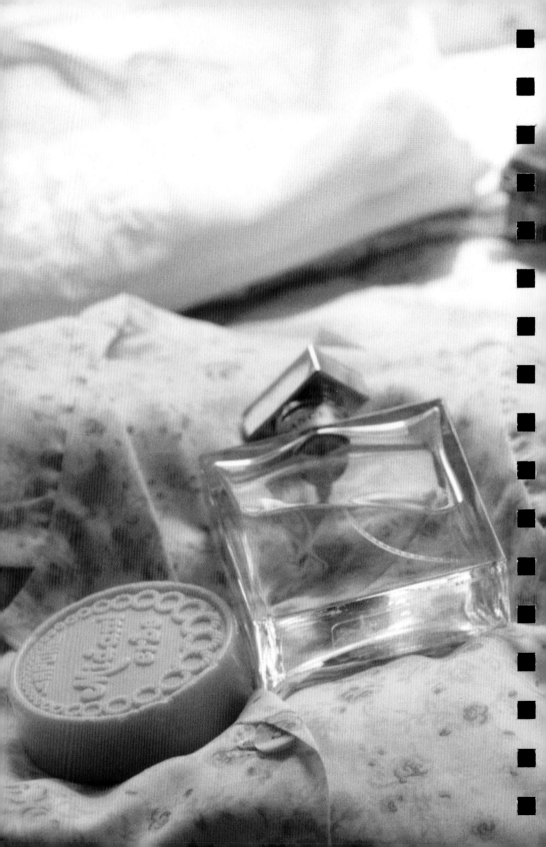

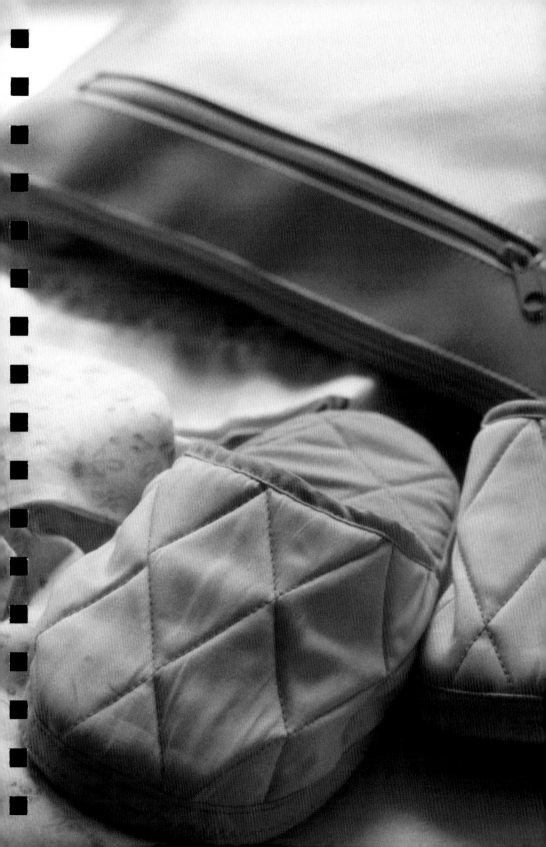

week 38

you

at about this time you may feel your fundus 'drop' as the fetal head descends or 'engages' in the pelvis. This is also accompanied by an increased sensation of pressure in the lower abdomen and pelvic floor. If it is your first pregnancy, this is more likely to happen at this stage; engagement is more likely to be closer to term in subsequent pregnancies. If this does not happen, it may indicate that there is some disproportion between the size of the pelvis and the presenting part of the baby, or that there is some other obstruction, such as a low-lying placenta, a fibroid or an ovarian cyst. An ultrasound examination may be worthwhile at this stage to exclude these possibilities. A pelvic CT scan to assess the size and shape of the birth canal may also be of value.

MY WEIGHT _____

MY BELLY WIDTH _____

APPOINTMENTS _____

week 38

your baby

if you do not feel any movements for a day or if there is a dramatic rather than a gradual change in the nature of these movements, contact your doctor or the hospital so that the fetal condition can be checked. This check may involve a fetal heart rate trace or CTG, which assesses the fetal heart rate in relation to fetal movement and uterine activity. This can provide valuable information about the fetal condition.

Your baby measures 50 cm (19.7 in) and weighs 3.1 kg (6.8 lb).

baby clothes

During her first year, your baby will grow amazingly fast. Don't buy too many clothes as she will outgrow a complete wardrobe about every two to three months. Friends and family will also buy clothes as gifts for the newborn baby. If someone asks you what you would like as a gift for baby, consider a gift voucher as you can use this during the months to come when baby has outgrown her first wardrobe. If you are uncomfortable with this, ask for clothes for three-, six-, nine- and 12-month-old babies.

Suggested list of baby clothes

- 3 nighties
- 6 all-in-one stretch suits with crotch opening
- 6 singlets
- 6 pairs of pilchers
- 2 cardigans or tops
- 4 pairs of bootees or socks
- 3 or 4 cotton bunny rugs
- 1 sun hat

For winter

- 2 bonnets or warm hats
- 1 warm shawl
- 2 sleeping bags
- 2 woollen jumpers or cardigans

notes _____

_____

_____

_____

_____

_____

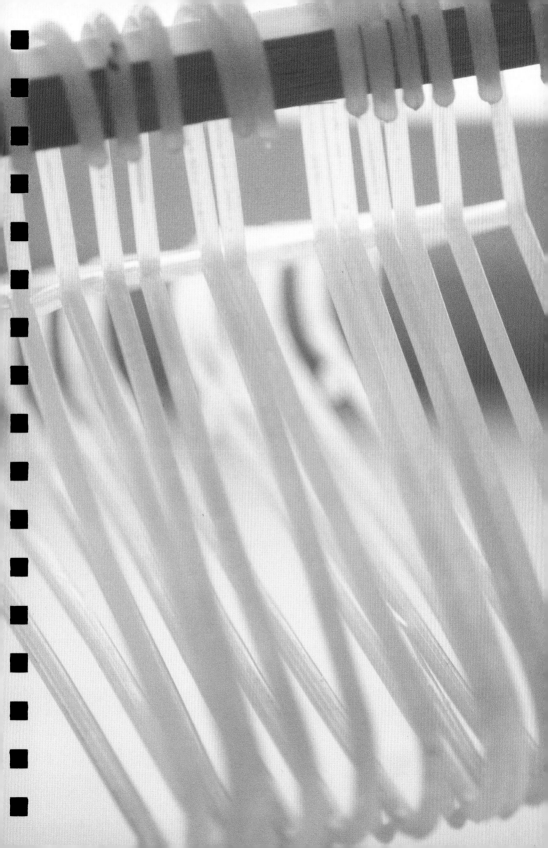

DATE . . . .

you

your pregnancy is now considered to be at term as the baby normally delivers between 38 and 42 weeks. You are no doubt becoming increasingly impatient, not to mention a little apprehensive, about the imminent birth. One or two of the following signs marks the onset of true labour: the commencement of regular uterine contractions that may be painful, the passage of a small amount of sticky, bloodstained mucus from the vagina (the 'show') and gushing of amniotic fluid from the vagina, signifying rupture of the membranes. Labour generally starts within 24 hours of the 'show'. If labour does not start within 24 hours of your membranes rupturing, your doctor may consider inducing contractions with oxytocin or prostaglandins.

It is not clear why labour starts in the human but it is most likely a combination of your baby, your uterus and the prostaglandins secreted by the membranes. Premature labour and ruptured membranes may be the result of infection spreading up from the vagina through the cervix. Intercourse may precipitate labour in late pregnancy as semen is rich in prostaglandins, which cause the uterus to contract; however, the uterus must be ready to start contracting in order for this to occur.

Obstetricians sometimes 'strip the membranes' while doing an internal examination in order to start labour, as this also releases prostaglandins.

MY WEIGHT _____

MY BELLY WIDTH _____

APPOINTMENTS _____

APPROXIMATELY 10 DAYS TO GO

your baby now measures over 51 cm (20 in) and weighs around 3.3 kg (7.3 lb); however, do remember that babies vary enormously in size, with the normal range extending from 2.5 kg (5.5 lb) to 4.5 kg (10 lb). As a rule, boys are slightly heavier than girls by an average of 100 g (3.5 oz).

your baby

DATE ....

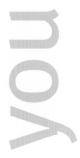

when labour has commenced it is important to go to the hospital where you are booked for delivery. As early labour can take a long time, particularly in your first pregnancy, try not to go in too soon. It is often better to remain mobile at home at this early stage although you should discuss this with your delivery team at the time. As subsequent labours tend to be more efficient and shorter, you should probably avoid staying at home in later pregnancies.

When the time has finally come and you are in 'true' labour, you should make your way to the hospital with your packed labour kit and hospital bag. If possible, wash your hair and do your nails before you leave home, as you never know when you will get the opportunity to perform these essential tasks again and you will want to look your best for the photos following the delivery. Interestingly, this grooming behaviour is more common before the first birth than for subsequent ones.

MY WEIGHT

MY BELLY WIDTH

APPOINTMENTS

APPROXIMATELY 3 DAYS TO GO

your baby

the baby's skin is now smooth and the fine lanugo hair, which previously covered it entirely, is now largely confined to the shoulders. The skin is still covered by the greasy vernix caseosa, which both facilitates the birth process and helps keep the baby warm after delivery. The baby's head is also covered by a varying amount of hair. The skull bones are now somewhat firmer, although the gaps between them (the fontanelles) are still open. The one at the front can be felt as a soft diamond-shaped depression and the one at the back is a Y-shaped groove. These allow the obstetrician or midwife to determine the position of the head during labour.

The head is now in proportion to the body, measuring approximately one-quarter of the body's length. The eyes are open, the nose is well formed and the ears stand out from the head. The genitals are also well formed and in the male fetus the testes should be in the scrotum.

Your baby weighs 3.5 kg (7.7 lb) and measures 52 cm (20.4 in).

Your baby is as large as... **a newborn**

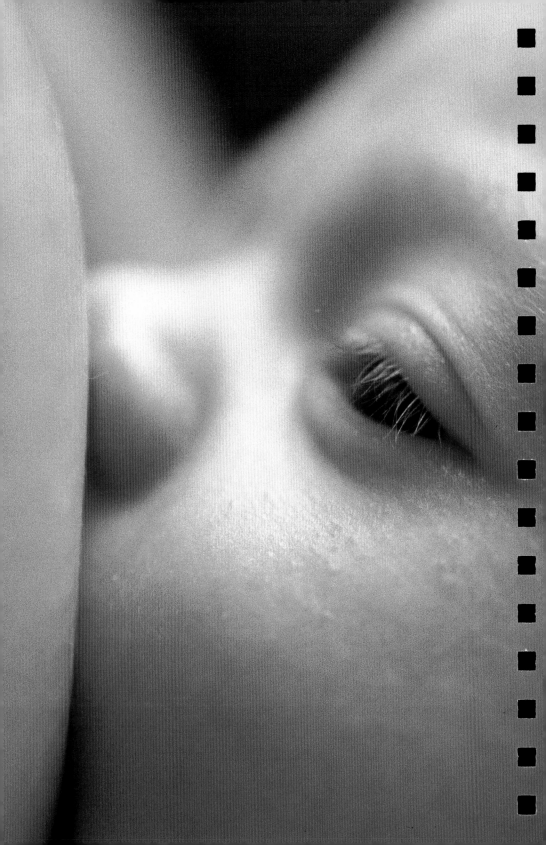

feeding baby

Feeding the baby is the first major issue you'll confront after the birth. Most women will have a view on the 'breast versus bottle' debate. This is an individual choice and will depend on a variety of cultural, familial, physical and emotional factors. But whether you decide to breast- or bottle-feed, there are a number of items you'll need.

Breastfeeding

- Breast pads
- 3 nursing bras
- Breast pump
- Sterilising kit
- Bottles for expressed milk

Bottle-feeding

- Baby milk formula
  (suitable for a newborn)
- 6–8 bottles, teats and covers
- Sterilising kit
- Bottle brush

notes _____

_____

_____

_____

_____

_____

_____

_____

_____

_____

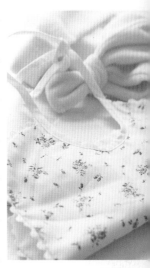

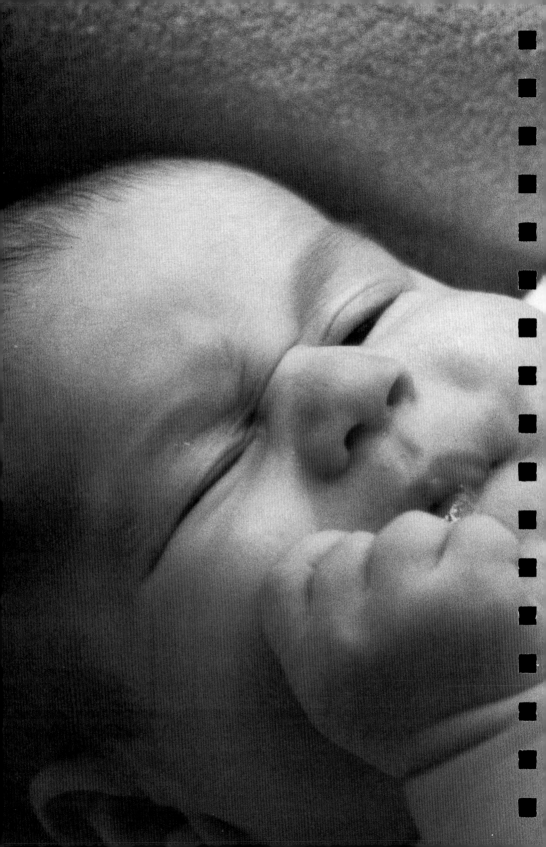

after the birth

congratulations
The pregnancy is over and your baby has finally arrived. The next 48 hours will be a blur of emotions, congratulations and new experiences.

week 1 (days 1–7)

you & your baby

introduction
Most women deliver their babies in hospital (only 1–2 per cent deliver at home) and approximately 20 per cent will deliver by caesarean section. So the hospital will be your first postnatal experience and the midwives will be your first educators in the long learning curve to becoming a competent parent.

bonding
The importance of bonding with your new baby cannot be overstated. The first few days of your baby's life, particularly the first few hours, are critical. Cuddle your baby as soon as you can after delivery. For mother and baby, it's an interchange of signs, signals, smells, caresses and sounds. This is when your baby identifies you as her mother. Hold and touch your baby as often as you can, make eye contact, speak and sing to her. When feeding, smile at her and talk to her. Let your baby touch your skin, which will automatically happen when you're breastfeeding.

This is the time when you will begin to interpret your baby's signals. Watch how she tells you she is hungry, tired or needs changing. If you concentrate on interpreting these signs in the first few days, you will reap the rewards when you go home from hospital. If your baby is in the hospital nursery due to premature delivery or for another reason, spend as much time as you can in the nursery, touching her and talking to her. Insist on being able to do this.

breastfeeding
On each nipple there are between six and 15 openings from the lactiferous ducts and sinuses draining each lobe of the breast. Colostrum is the 'pre-milk' that can be secreted late in pregnancy and in the first two to three days after delivery. It is yellowish, thick and high in protein, and contains antibodies to help the baby's immune system.

week 1 (days 1–7)

The true milk 'comes in' at around day 3. One gram (0.04 oz) of breast tissue produces 1–2 g (0.04–0.07 oz) of milk per day. Suckling induces the brain to produce a chemical (oxytocin) that forces the milk into the lactiferous sinuses just under the areola. This is called the 'let-down' reflex. This chemical also helps the uterus contract and reduces bleeding. The baby obtains most of the available milk in the first few minutes if her mouth is properly attached — both the areola and the nipple should be in her mouth. Poor positioning can make 'latching on' difficult and can cause cracked nipples. Prolonged suckling can also result in cracked nipples and 'air swallowing'. Emptying the breasts (manually if necessary) can prevent painful engorgement in the first week.

Breastfeeding is an energy-sapping business and it is vital to eat well and drink plenty of water. Remember that many of the things you eat and drink end up in the breastmilk, so be cautious with drugs (including alcohol and nicotine) and certain foods that may upset the baby's digestive system (typically spicy foods and peas!).

support person If you have had a caesarean section, ask the hospital if your support person or relative can stay in the hospital overnight for a couple of days. Most private hospitals and some public hospitals allow this. It probably won't be necessary on the first night following the operation, as hospital staff will monitor you closely. Because nursing staff are very busy and your caesarean wound could be painful for a few days, it might be very helpful to have your partner or a friend help you with showering, getting to the toilet, passing baby to you or simply fetching items from drawers or bags.

week 1 (days 1–7)

you & your baby

how you feel
Exhaustion dominates everything for the first couple of days as you recover from the enormous physical exertions of labour and learn to cope with disturbed sleep. It is important to *rest* when you can.

A burst of emotions will sweep you along for the first few days — relief that your baby is normal, joy at the new arrival and anxiety regarding the tasks and hurdles ahead. Many women experience early 'blues' due to pain, fatigue, lack of attention, feeding difficulties, hormonal changes, and unspoken worries and fears. This is usually transient, but in a small number of women it can persist for weeks or months as postnatal depression.

early physical changes
The uterus is 20 cm (7.9 in) long after delivery (the size of a rock melon) and weighs around 1 kg (2.2 lb), but it reduces to the size of a grapefruit by the end of the first week. It keeps contracting for 12–24 hours after delivery and can create mild 'after-pains'. Blood loss from the placental site in the first three to four days is dark red (lochia rubra) and like a very heavy period. Loss of more than 500 mL (0.9 pt) blood is called a postpartum hemorrhage. This can occur within the first 24 hours after delivery (when it is called primary) or from day 2 to 42 hours (called secondary).

Perineal healing is rapid and often complete by day 5 (dissolvable sutures or stitches are exclusively used for repair of tears or episiotomies). This healing process is aided by frequent showers (remember not to use powder as it is uncomfortable and can slow healing if it enters the wound). If you have an abdominal caesarean section wound, this will require daily dressings for the first day or two and can be left open from day 3. These sutures are also usually dissolvable.

week 1 (days 1–7)

You'll pass an enormous amount of urine in the first few days. This will get rid of the body water (oedema) which has accumulated during your pregnancy. You may also experience constipation. This is common in new mothers, whose fear of the pain accompanying bowel movements may make the problem worse. You can prevent constipation by drinking lots of water, having an adequate fibre intake and also by taking simple laxatives if necessary. Try prunes, fruit, muesli or liquorice, or a good proprietary laxative.

Be alert for signs of deep vein thrombosis, such as a painful, swollen leg. You are at greater risk if you are older, overweight or have had an operative delivery (caesarean section or forceps). You can reduce this risk by getting up and moving around as soon as possible after the birth as well as by drinking plenty of water. In higher risk situations you may be given subcutaneous injections of the blood-thinning agent, heparin.

Look for any signs of infection. The most likely sites are the perineum, uterus, breast and bladder. Infection anywhere can cause an increase in temperature. Infection in the perineum causes pain and swelling at the site; infection in the bladder makes you urinate frequently and causes pain on urination; and in the uterus it causes an offensive vaginal discharge and a tender uterus.

postnatal exercises Start doing the recommended postnatal exercises in hospital or as soon as you feel comfortable doing so. Back and pelvic floor exercises are very important for strengthening muscles and ligaments that have been stretched during pregnancy. They are good for getting your figure back quickly too. Ask the hospital staff for information.

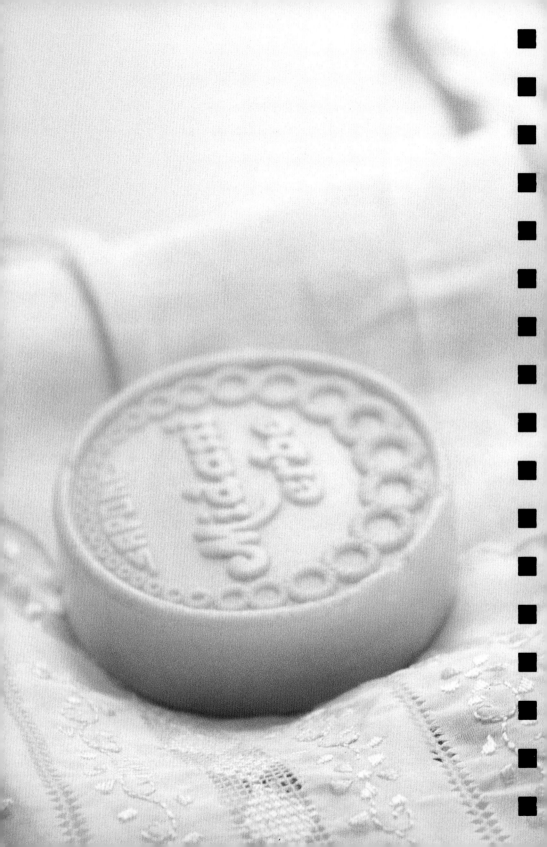

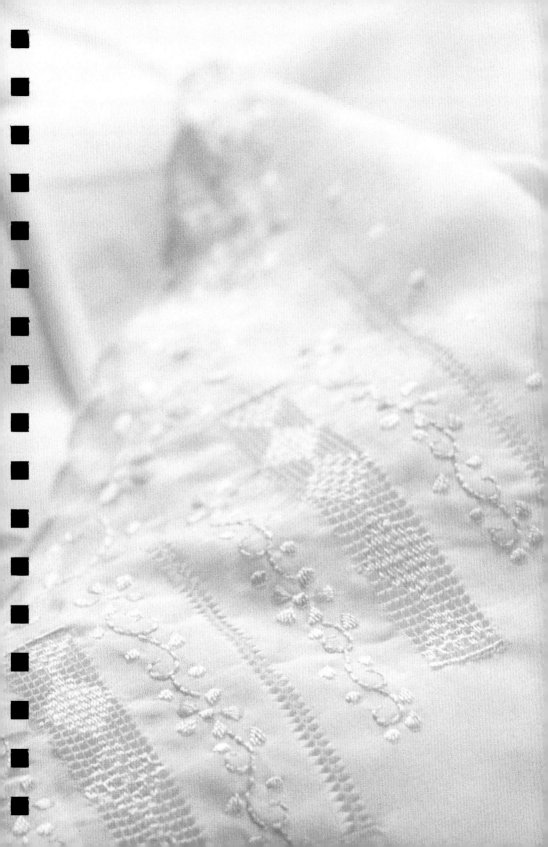

week 1 (days 1–7)

your baby In this first week your baby is also undergoing rapid changes. The average birth weight for a full-term baby is 3.5 kg (7.7 lb). Loss of up to 10 per cent of the birth weight is not uncommon in the first week. Ninety-eight per cent of babies are structurally normal. A pediatrician will quickly review the baby at birth to exclude major problems and will more thoroughly assess the baby in the next 48 hours (or prior to your discharge from hospital). Newborn screening, to exclude a number of rare genetic syndromes such as cystic fibrosis and phenylketonuria, is performed on day 5 on blood obtained by heel-prick. The baby usually has an injection of vitamin K in the first day or two to prevent certain bleeding disorders.

Mild jaundice occurs in many babies in the first few days after birth, because the liver has not started to operate fully and some blood products tend to accumulate in the tissues. This is called physiological jaundice. It usually settles in a day or two without any specific intervention, but occasionally the baby will need to be placed under ultraviolet light, which increases the metabolism of these products and helps to resolve the jaundice. Other forms of jaundice that are due to blood group incompatibility sometimes require more intensive treatment, but thankfully they are quite uncommon. Jaundiced babies tend to become sleepy and thence dehydrated as they do not suck. If your baby is jaundiced you may be asked to keep her well fed and hydrated by feeding her more frequently.

In the first few hours after birth your baby is likely to breathe rapidly. In the first few days she may have white 'pimples' (milia) on the nose and cheeks, mild jaundice and enlarged breasts. These are mostly changes that resolve themselves, requiring no specific treatment. The umbilical cord stump usually dries

week 1 (days 1–7)

(assisted by normal washing in bathwater and a daily application of methylated spirits with a cotton bud if it becomes smelly) and drops off after a few days.

You can start breastfeeding as soon as practicable after delivery. It is common for baby to bring up a little milk/colostrum (posset) along with 'wind' after each feed. Baby's first bowel motion, called meconium, is almost black as well as sticky but subsequent motions are green, brown, then yellow with 'mustard seeds' in it due to the milk curd after five to six days. If you bottle-feed your baby, her poo will reach the brown stage sooner, as she does not have to wait for your breastmilk to come in.

settling baby If baby is unsettled and having a bad day, she may be having a growth spurt and needs more milk. At these times you can offer her a supplement or use some stored expressed milk. You produce breastmilk on a supply and demand basis. The more your baby needs, the more you will produce, but it can take a couple of days to increase the supply. Offer your baby more feeds during the day to build up your supply and make sure you drink more water at these times.

Taking a cranky baby for a walk in the pram or stroller will nearly always settle her down. The fresh air and change of scene is great for you and the baby, and there is the beneficial side effect of the exercise you get.

The nursing staff at the hospital will teach you how to wrap your baby in order to settle her for a sleep. Wrapping your baby will prevent her from jerking herself awake during REM sleep. This technique may include wrapping her arms although some babies prefer to have their arms free. Your early childhood nurse or

you & your baby

health visitor can also advise you on how to wrap your baby. You will need to make an appointment with her within one week of being discharged from hospital: she will be a wealth of information and support.

Having a new baby in the house and suffering the associated sleep deprivation will inevitably make you feel tired, uptight and stressed. A crying baby will tend to exacerbate these feelings. Your baby can sense how you feel and may be unsettled by it. When you are breastfeeding or in bed at night, do some of the relaxation exercises you learnt in antenatal classes. Take three deep breaths and relax. Try taking on a calm demeanour even if you don't feel calm. It will help you, even if it doesn't fool your baby.

If your baby is very unsettled and you are feeling as if you are not coping, call your local mothercraft centre. The counsellor you speak to on the phone may suggest you make an appointment for a consultation. You may eventually be advised to stay overnight so the staff there can assess the problems and design a regimen for you and your baby. *Never* be afraid to ask for help!

visitors
After the birth, well-meaning friends and family can create an unending stream of visitors in hospital. This can be exhausting, especially as you will be recovering from your delivery. You could suggest that friends wait until the second day to visit, explaining that the first day is for family.

postnatal depression
About three days after having your baby you can expect to feel a bit down, to cry and feel sad. The 'blues' are due to the sudden change in hormone levels in your body. Accept that this is happening to your body,

and tell your partner and hospital staff. The feeling usually passes in a day or so. If these feelings persist or return after you have gone home, you may have postnatal depression.

These are the warning signs for postnatal depression.

- Feeling alone
- Not enjoying your baby
- Feeling sad most of the time
- Feelings of inadequacy
- Crying easily for no obvious reason
- Experiencing a lack of energy or enthusiasm
- Thinking nobody understands how you are feeling
- Not sleeping well, even when you get the opportunity
- Feeling anxious, worried, irritable
- Being unable to see a solution to your problem

It's vital that you speak to your early childhood clinic nurse or family doctor as soon as possible. You can also phone support services (see the list of support groups on page 189). Remember that help is readily available.

going home
How soon after the birth you will go home will depend on the type of delivery; your own wishes, level of confidence and support; and the health of you and your baby. Some discussion about contraception is appropriate (although sex may be the farthest thing from your mind at the moment!). Ovulation can occur as early as three weeks after delivery if you are not breastfeeding (and remember, breastfeeding is *not* an adequate contraceptive).

spending time with your toddler

Having a new baby in the house can be very demanding. It is impossible to devote the same amount of time and attention to a toddler that you did before the new baby's arrival.

Once you settle the new baby for a sleep, you may be sorely tempted to rush around and do loads of washing or other household chores. But it's very important to spend a little of this time with your toddler. He will be feeling neglected and craving some time alone with you. Have a little game or activity prepared, or simply sit and cuddle your toddler and chat with him. You could then ask him to help you: if you're putting washing on the line, ask him to pass the pegs and name their colours as he goes.

When you are feeding or bathing the baby, your toddler will soon learn that he can get your attention — albeit negative attention — by being naughty. It's much better to keep him occupied during these times.

When breastfeeding (or bottle-feeding) the new baby, read to your toddler. At baby's bathtime, ask him to help by passing you nappies, creams, baby's hairbrush or clothes. However, if he is too young, it may be better to settle your toddler with his favourite video or television show.

On the weekend, ask your partner to look after the baby for a couple of hours so that you can spend some special time with your toddler or older children.

A walk to the local park with baby in the pram can be a lovely outing for everyone — and it doesn't cost anything!

Grandparents are wonderful at making a special fuss of toddlers. It may be a special treat to let your child spend a night at his grandparents' house — just to be spoilt.

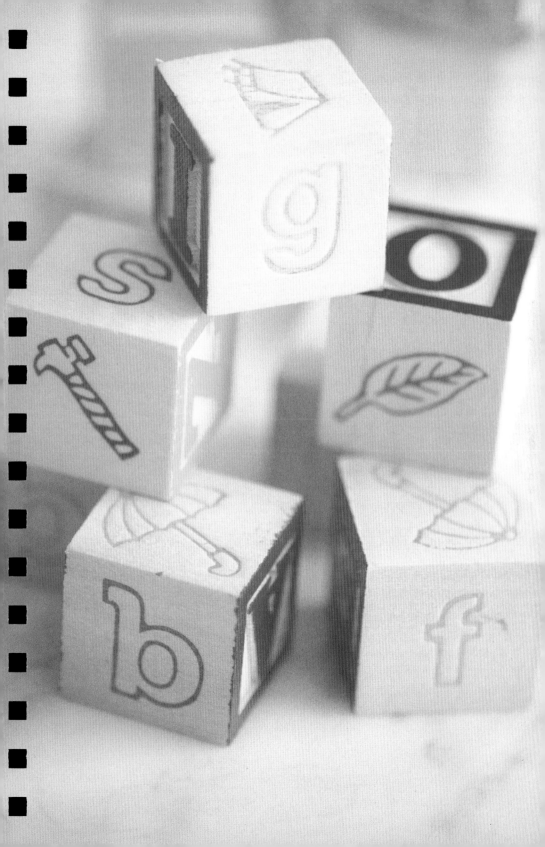

week 2 (days 8–14)

DATE ....

home again Now you're back at home, enlist all the help you can with daily household chores so that you can concentrate on yourself and your baby. This is probably the best week for your partner to take time off, both as an emotional support during this transition/learning phase and as a physical support to keep the household running. (A vital part of antenatal planning is housetraining your partner if he is not already reasonably domesticated!)

Tiredness is still the governing feature in your life but just being back in your own environment will probably give you a tremendous lift. Learn to be relaxed with your baby — don't jump out of your skin with every murmur! This week is all about developing a routine that suits you both, whether you are feeding, resting, bathing or playing.

how you feel The physical changes affecting you this week are less dramatic than last week. The dark red blood loss has given way to a thinner and paler discharge (lochia serosa), which then reduces to the thicker lochia alba. Your blood pressure should be back to normal by now. Your breasts are generally becoming more comfortable, while your nipples become pliant and soft. Breast engorgement is less common by now. Weakening of the pelvic floor is common after childbirth and may influence bowel and bladder security: start gentle pelvic floor exercises this week if you haven't already done so.

your baby Your newborn is ruled by hunger at this stage, with sleep running a close second. She will need to be fed every three to four hours around the clock. Most babies will sleep for 17–18 hours in a 24-hour period. Your baby will move in and out of several states of sleepiness, quiet alertness and active

you & your baby

week 2 (days 8–14)

alertness. It's never too early to start the learning process. In the few moments of quiet wakefulness, stimulate your baby's senses with bright objects and mobiles, and play with a variety of sounds. Gentle massage and passive limb movements are soothing for your baby.

At this stage of your newborn's development, the 'primitive' reflexes dominate. These are the grasp reflex (when a baby curls her fingers around an object touching her palm) and the stepping reflex (when you hold baby up and touch her feet on a surface she appears to try to walk). Your baby is not yet capable of purposeful limb or head movements.

week 3 (days 15–21)

you & your baby

out and about Now that your confidence is building, it's time to get out and about and show off your baby. The next challenge to consider is 'baby on the move' — weigh up the pros and cons of slings and capsules, prams and strollers (the lying down variety at this stage). Your choice will depend on the destination and your mode of transport. Think about your back; your baby will get heavier very quickly so good quality equipment is worth the investment (see page 166 for advice).

diet It's important not to neglect your diet. Eat plenty of carbohydrates (bread, cereal, pasta), protein-rich foods (red meat, oily fish), fruit and vegetables. Moderate amounts of milk and dairy foods are beneficial but eat fats and simple sugars sparingly. Try to maintain a high fluid intake, especially if you are breastfeeding. You should aim to drink 2–3 L (3.5–5.3 pt) of water a day. Keep your tea and coffee intake down as it has a dehydrating effect on you and the caffeine may upset your baby.

exercise Your prepregnancy flat tummy will not have returned just yet, but doing some gentle postnatal exercises will improve general tone and your feeling of wellbeing. Doing this with a group of other new mothers helps you to feel motivated; most gyms have postnatal exercise and aqua-aerobic classes. Many bigger gyms also have a crèche or baby-minding facilities.

your baby Your newborn doesn't seem to have much of a personality at this stage, and mainly expresses herself by crying. However, she will respond to sound, lift her head when placed on her tummy and stare at faces (or her own in a mirror). The newborn's vision is thought to be 'fuzzy' so she is able to focus only on close objects, such as your face when you are feeding her.

week 3 (days 15–21)

getting organised Sometimes simply getting into the shower and out of your dressing gown before noon can be a challenge. Try to shower and dress before your partner leaves the house for the day. Even if you get back into bed for a while, you'll feel ready for your day when the baby wakes.

adjustments After the initial excitement of your baby's arrival, life takes on a whole new dimension, and after a few weeks, it is common for your partner to feel a little neglected. He no longer has all your attention; in fact, he probably has very little. The house has no doubt been a bit chaotic and your attention has been absorbed by the new person in your home. Even though it will take some extra effort, prepare a special dinner or order a takeaway meal.

If you can't arrange for a babysitter for a couple of hours, simply settle the baby and wait until she is asleep. You could even light a couple of candles, and enjoy dinner and talking to each other — just like you used to before your baby was born. Try not to talk about the baby unless your partner wants to. It's easy to forget about romance but it's so important that you don't!

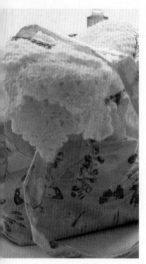

for outings
If you shop wisely for these items you'll be rewarded with lasting service.

- **Pram/stroller** Once again, make sure the pram/stroller you select is the right height. You will spend many hours behind this piece of equipment and it will be unsatisfactory if you have to bend over to push it or if the handles are uncomfortably high for you.

  Select a strong, stable pram with an easy to use harness and frame locks. A built-in shopping bag or tray is always useful. Never hang shopping bags on the handles of the pram as they will destabilise it, causing it to overturn. Before you buy a pram, make sure it conforms to the relevant standard. It's also a good idea to buy a pram with a storm cover, just in case you are caught in the rain.

- **Baby car seat or capsule** You will need to buy or hire a baby capsule and have it properly fitted to your car before you take your baby home from hospital. Either organise this before you go into labour or get your partner to do it while you're still in hospital. Some hospitals have a special fitting service on site.

- **Slings and backpacks** Slings or backpacks are a great way to transport baby when strollers are impractical but don't forget the baby sunscreen and sun hat. A baby's skin is very sensitive to the sun.

- **Baby's bag** Always have a bag packed with all your baby's needs — change of clothes, nappies, wipes, pilchers, creams and toys — ready for the next outing. Buy, or make, a large bag or nappy bag, as they are usually known. A waterproof change mat is a handy item to keep in this bag. You'll be surprised how many times you'll need to change baby's nappy in an awkward place, and your own waterproof mat will ensure that you always have a clean surface for this purpose.

- **Portable cot** While portable cots can be expensive, they are handy for overnight stays and holidays, especially if you'll be leaving baby with friends or relatives. As your baby becomes familiar with the cot, you'll find it easier to settle her when she is away from home.

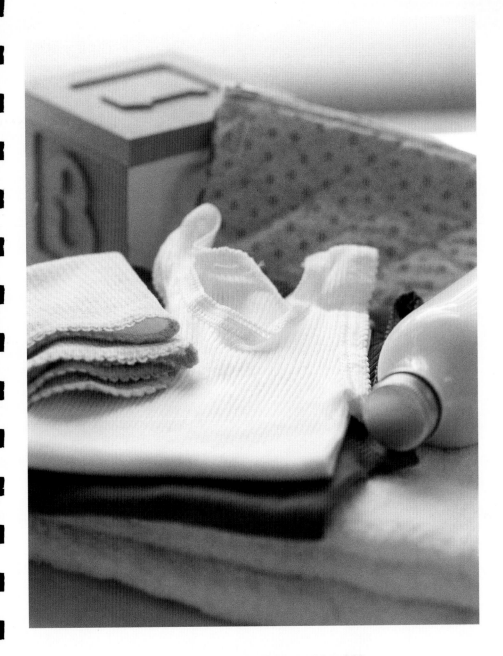

You can leave it in the car so you're always prepared for visiting.
Choose a portable cot that conforms to the appropriate standard.
Check that the mattress supplied with the cot fits snugly all the way
around and that any mechanisms for collapsing the cot are easy
for you to use but hard for a child to operate.

week 4 (days 22–28)

gaining confidence
You've now established a routine that allows you to achieve all the baby care tasks to be achieved (and, sadly, you can also fit in household chores). You are confidently managing tasks that you approached with anxiety only a couple of weeks ago.

pacing yourself
You do get used to coping with broken sleep, but it takes its toll. Make sure you program in some recovery time for yourself during the day. When the baby goes down for a sleep during the day it's a good idea to put your feet up and read or snooze. Don't worry too much about the housework — it will still be there later. It's much better to feel rested and able to cope than to have a spotless house.

socialising
Don't become so focused on your baby that you end up isolated at home. Stay involved with your mothers' group, family and friends (especially those with young children who will have a greater understanding of the highs and lows you're experiencing).

how you feel
For most women the vaginal (lochial) discharge should stop this week. Breast and nipple discomfort has usually settled by now (unless your baby decides on a longer than usual sleep and you're suddenly full to overflowing). Gradually increase your level of physical activity. Try to walk with your baby in a pram or stroller every day, or swim when you can. Don't worry about weight loss or dietary restrictions at this stage. Your baby will 'eat the weight off you', despite what you may think is a huge intake of food (you need an extra 20–30 per cent energy intake per day just to keep up with the demands of breastfeeding her).

week 4 (days 22–28)

your baby

Your baby suddenly seems to be expanding in all directions. She will have added nearly 1 kg (2.2 lb) to her birth weight and is about 4 cm (1.6 in) longer by the end of the first month. All of a sudden those size oo sleepsuits seem very inadequate! Your baby has reached her peak breastmilk intake during this week (around 550 mL or 1 pt per day or 190 g/kg — that is, 0.42 lb/2.2 lb — body weight per day).

Your baby also seems to be interacting more with the environment: her head and eyes follow objects. It is important to get to know your baby. Set aside some time when the baby is content and just look at each other. You may notice her staring at your face quite intently. Research shows that babies can see black and white patterns, and some behaviourists suggest babies of this age are 'mapping' your features so they can recognise you. Whatever is actually going on, it's a lovely bonding experience and a nice break from the hurly-burly of 'new baby' life.

housework

You won't have much time for cleaning with a new baby in the house and as long as the baby's room, the bathroom and the kitchen are clean, the rest can wait. It's amazing how little housework is necessary when time and energy are the deciding factors. A spare room is a godsend: tidy the house in minutes by throwing everything into this room if visitors are about to arrive.

If friends or family members ask if they can help in any way, accept the offer! Ask them to clean the floors, put some washing on the line or do the shopping. People really do want to help. Remember, your baby will grow up fast. Forget the housework and enjoy your baby. If you have the choice of cleaning the oven or giving your baby a cuddle, cuddle the baby!

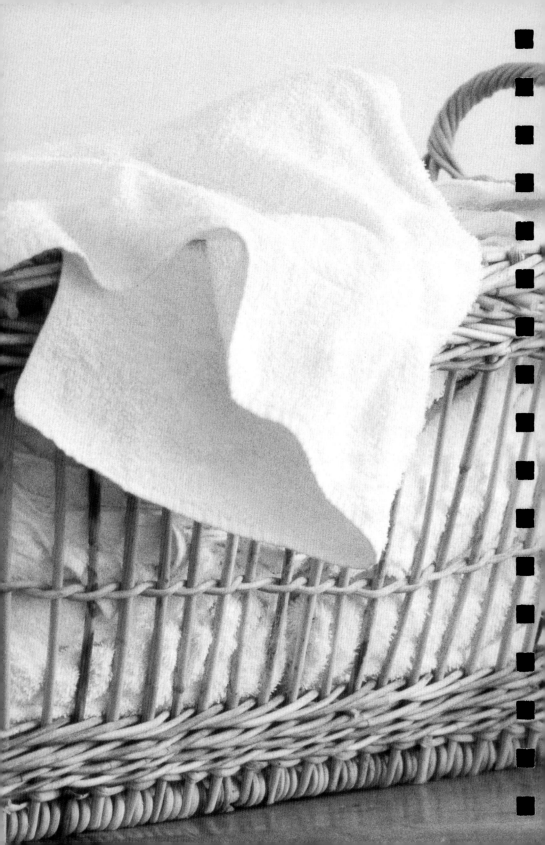

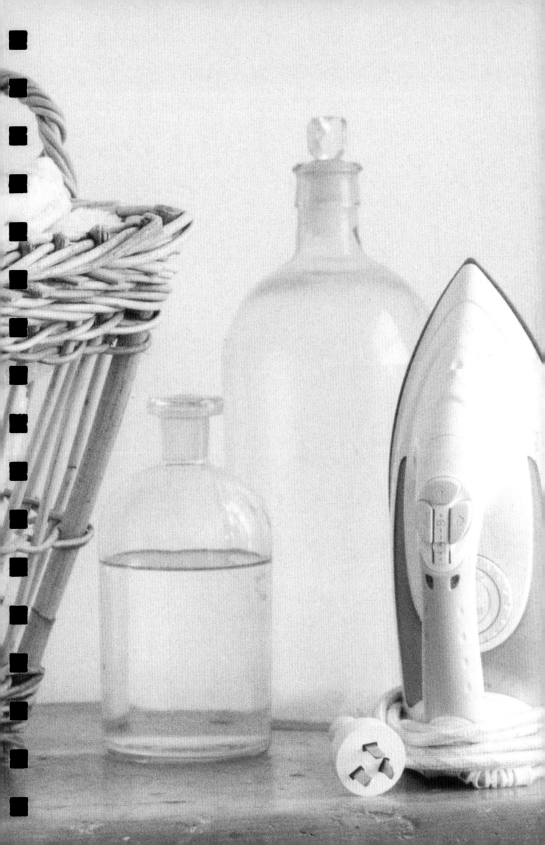

week 5 (days 29–35)

you & your baby

your sexuality

As the vaginal discharge diminishes and your routine is hopefully allowing adequate rest, you may be rediscovering your sexuality. Any interest in sexual activity is heavily influenced by tiredness and the presence of persistent vaginal loss or perineal discomfort. It is natural to feel some anxiety about sex at this time; your partner will need to be gentle and cooperative.

This is a good time to review the contraceptive issue, if you haven't already. Remember that breastfeeding alone is not an effective contraceptive. Many couples use condoms until they make a decision about the timing of a future pregnancy. The most efficient method while breastfeeding (other than abstinence) is the 'mini-pill'. This only contains progesterone, which does not interfere with the breastmilk supply. Some women will elect to breastfeed for three to six months and then return to the combined pill once the baby has been weaned. Intra-uterine contraceptive devices are not appropriate in the first six weeks after delivery. The choice is yours; you may want to discuss the issue with your obstetrician or family doctor at the first postnatal visit next week.

your baby

Your baby seems to be doing more all of a sudden. Along with the soulful stares, there are now smiles and laughs and plenty of rewarding gurgles and 'oohs and aahs'. Lots of head and limb movements are happening (without too much coordination at this stage). Your baby will love being carried around in a front pack or sling so she is warm and close to you — the added bonus is that you have two free hands!

week 5 (days 29–35)

toning and stretching
A timely reminder...look after your back. The ligaments supporting your spine and pelvis were softened and stretched due to the action of progesterone during the pregnancy. These are now returning to normal but the muscle strength and tone may still not be as good as they were before pregnancy. This can be compounded by all the lifting and other postural demands of looking after your baby. Take a little time each day to do some toning and stretching exercises. Exercising with a large inflatable ball is useful for abdominal and back strengthening, but check with a gym instructor or physiotherapist first and ask him or her to design an exercise program for you. Swim if you can.

week 6 (days 36–42)

you & your baby

settling into motherhood

You've survived the first six weeks. You should take some time to reflect on that short but very steep learning curve (now that you're comfortably nearing the top of it!). You are entitled to be impressed by your transition from 'nervous newby' to competent parent. This is the end of the puerperal phase — the period after birth when tradition suggests that everything is back to normal (although in this postdelivery world you may not be sure what normal is any more).

postnatal visit

This week arrange a postnatal visit to your obstetrician (or family doctor or midwife). She will perform a general check-up, including blood pressure, perineal or abdominal wound healing check and a vaginal examination to ensure that the uterus has appropriately reduced in size (it should now weigh 100 g (3.5 oz) — about twice its prepregnant weight). This will also be an opportunity to perform a Pap smear if you haven't had one for two years or more.

first period

The placental site within the uterus has finally been covered over. This, along with the fact that the ovaries have returned to relatively normal hormone function, means that your first period often occurs in this week, even if you are breastfeeding. The first period is commonly heavy with clots, and is something of a rude shock. The red blood cell and hemoglobin levels should be back to prepregnant levels and you can generally stop taking iron tablets if you were anemic after delivery. Your heart rate has finally also returned to prepregnant levels (your heart having increased its rate and workload by up to 30 per cent during the pregnancy).

week 6 (days 36–42)

baby's check-up The early childhood centre mid-wives or your health visitor have kept a close eye on your baby's growth and development so far. If everything has been going well you probably haven't taken your baby to see your pediatrician (or family doctor) yet. This is an appropriate time to arrange a check-up for your baby. Your doctor will assess the baby's senses (sight and hearing) and reflexes, the heart (as many subtle changes aren't obvious at birth) and other organs, and check the hips for stability. Now is your chance to ask all those niggling questions that have been bothering you over the past few weeks. Write them down when they occur to you and take the list with you.

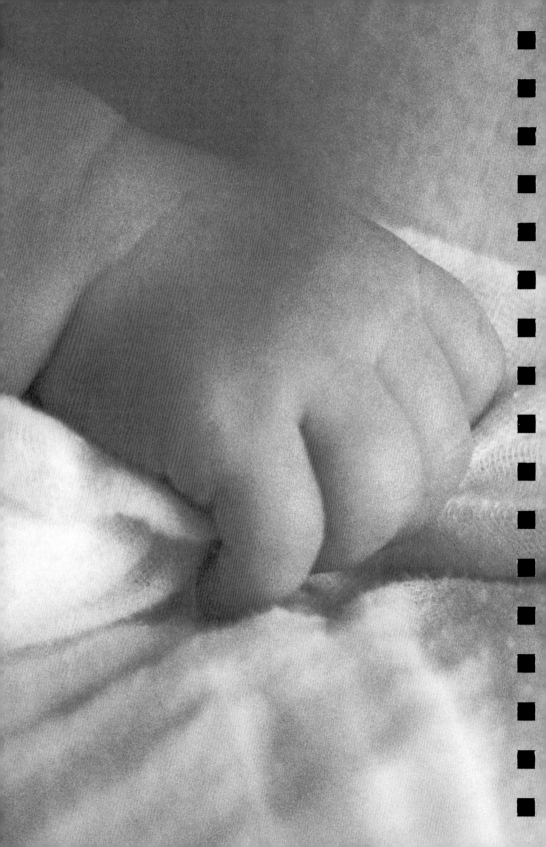

baby's journal

use these pages to record your baby's birth details and developmental milestones, to list the names of family and friends to contact after the birth, and to plan a christening or naming ceremony.

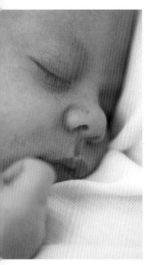

baby's arrival

name

born at

time

date

weight

head circumference

length

hair colour

my first thoughts

baby's development

first smiled

rolled onto back

slept all night

first tooth

first word

first step

age   weight   length

people to notify

name	telephone no.

name   telephone no.

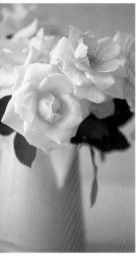

gifts received with thanks

_____

_____

_____

_____

_____

_____

_____

_____

_____

_____

_____

_____

_____

_____

planning christening/naming ceremony

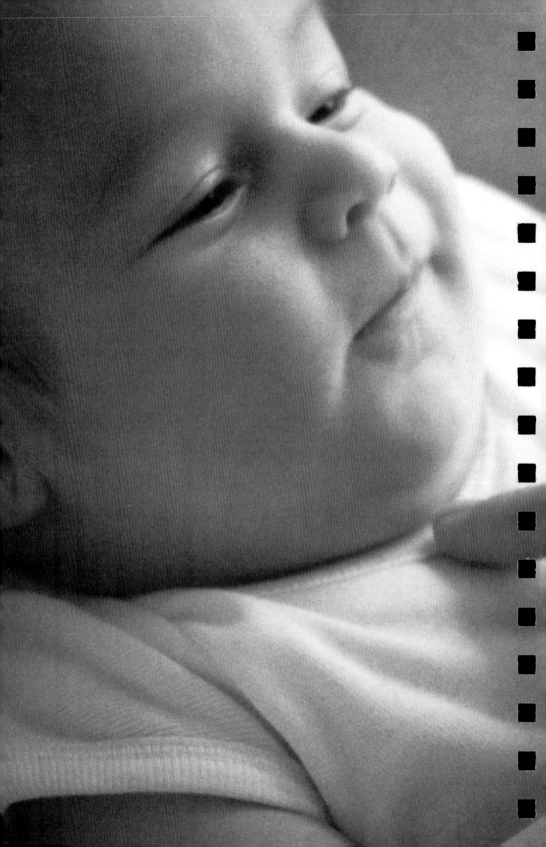

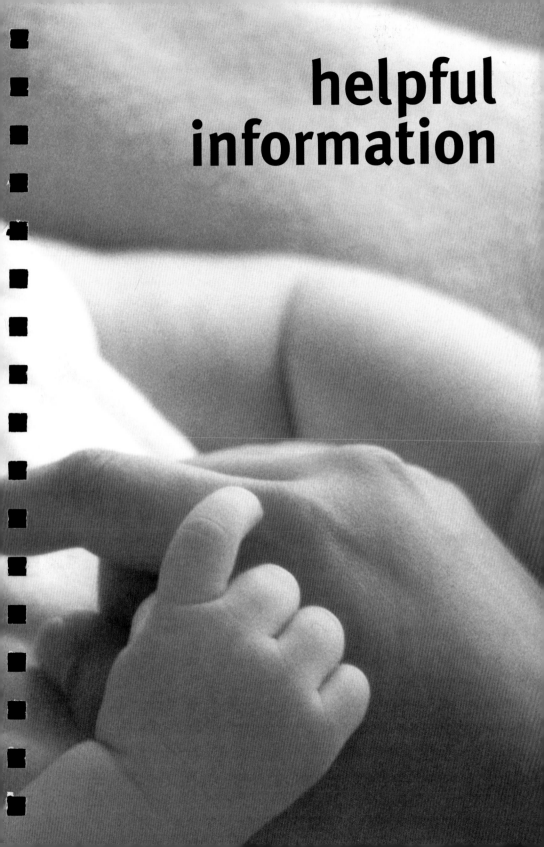

helpful information

medical terms

afterbirth the placenta and fetal membranes which are expelled from the uterus after birth

amniotic fluid waters surrounding the baby

amniotic membranes the membranes which enclose the amniotic fluid and its floating fetus. They protect the pregnancy from mechanical bumps and infections

antenatal before delivery of the baby

breech presentation bottom-first position of the baby in the uterus

cephalic head-first position of the baby in the uterus

EDC expected date of confinement

EDD expected date of delivery

embryo early fetus before it resembles a human (that is, up to about six weeks)

epidural spinal pain relief given to the mother during labour

fetus baby before birth

fundus top of the uterus

gestation duration of the pregnancy

LMP last menstrual period

placenta extraordinary organ responsible for the nutritional support of the baby throughout pregnancy. It weighs about 1.2 kg (2.6 lb) at birth

postnatal after delivery of the baby

umbilical cord tube through which oxygen and nourishment pass from the mother's placenta to the baby

uterus womb

vagina birth canal

support groups

You will find these support groups listed in your telephone directory.

Australia

Breastfeeding
Australian Breastfeeding Association
(formerly The Nursing Mother's
Association of Australia)

Multiple births
Australian Multiple Birth Association

Postnatal depression
PANDA (Post and Antenatal Depression
Association)

Single parents

NSW	Single Parent Family Association
	Solo Parents of Australia
	Parents Without Partners
VIC	Council for Single Mothers & Their Children
	Parents Without Partners
TAS	Family Support Service
	Parents Without Partners
QLD	Parents Without Partners
SA	Lone Parent Support Services
	SPARK Resource Centre
	Parents Without Partners
WA	Parents Without Partners

United Kingdom

Breastfeeding
Association of Breastfeeding Mothers
The Breastfeeding Network

Multiple births
Multiple Births Association (MBF)
Twins and Multiple Births Association
(TAMBA)

Postnatal depression
Association for Post Natal Illness
National Childbirth Trust

Single parents
Single and Custodial Fathers Network
Single Parents Association

index